Human Embryo Research: Yes or No?

Human Embryo Research:

YES OR NO?

THE CIBA FOUNDATION

Tavistock Publications
London and New York

First published in 1986
by Tavistock Publications
11 New Fetter Lane, London EC4P 4EE

Published in the USA by
Tavistock Publications
in association with Methuen, Inc.
29 West 35th Street, New York NY 10001

British Library Cataloguing in Publication Data

Human embryo research: yes or no?
1. Embryology, Human — Research
I. Ciba Foundation
612'.64'0072   QM601
ISBN 0-422-60590-5
ISBN 0-422-60600-6 Pbk

Library of Congress Cataloging in Publication Data

Human embryo research — yes or no?
Editors: Gregory Bock, Maeve O'Connor.
Papers from members of
a study group that met at the
Ciba Foundation on 6 and 7 Nov. 1985.
Includes bibliographies and indexes.
1. Human embryo — Research —
Moral and ethical aspects —Congresses.
I. Bock, Gregory. II. O'Connor, Maeve.
III. Ciba Foundation. [DNLM: 1. Abnormalities — congresses.
2. Embryology — congresses.
3. Fertilization in Vitro — congresses.
4. Infertility — congresses.
QS 620 H918 1985]
QM608.H85   1986   174.'28   86-14464
ISBN 0-422-60590-5
ISBN 0-422-60600-6 (pbk.)

Contents

Contributors

Members of a study group that met at the Ciba Foundation on 6 and 7 November, 1985. The idea for this study group was proposed by Dr Anne McLaren. The editors are Gregory Bock (Organizer) and Maeve O'Connor.

John Aitken, born in 1947, is a Senior Scientist with the MRC Unit of Reproductive Biology, and an Honorary Fellow of the Faculty of Medicine, University of Edinburgh. He is a scientific adviser to the World Health Organisation and in 1985 convened a meeting on behalf of WHO to discuss the role of interspecies *in vitro* fertilization in fertility diagnosis. His research interests lie in the molecular biology of human gametes, the application of such knowledge to the diagnosis and treatment of infertility, and the development of new approaches to contraception.

David Baird, born in 1935, is Professor of Obstetrics and Gynaecology, University of Edinburgh. He was a founder member of the MRC Unit of Reproductive Biology and continues as clinical adviser to the Centre for Reproductive Biology, University of Edinburgh. His research interests include the physiology of ovarian and menstrual cycles, and in recent years he has been consultant to a WHO Steering Committee on Infertility. He recently edited a book entitled *Mechanism of Menstruation*.

John Bowker, born in 1935, was Professor of Religious Studies, University of Lancaster from 1974 to 1985. He has been a member of commissions on religious education, doctrine, and marriage and divorce, and has edited and published books on comparative aspects of world religions. He is now Fellow and Dean of Chapel at Trinity College, Cambridge and adjunct professor at North Carolina State University, Raleigh, NC.

Peter Braude was born in South Africa in 1948. He is a member of the Royal College of Obstetricians and Gynaecologists, and holds a diploma in the Philosophy and Ethics of Medicine from the Society of Apothecaries. He is currently Senior Research Associate in the Department of Obstetrics and Gynaecology at the University of Cambridge and, with Dr Martin Johnson of the Anatomy Department, is co-holder of an MRC programme grant to investigate aspects of preimplantation development in mice and humans.

Peter Casey, born in 1948, is in the Science and Technology Secretariat of the Cabinet Office, working on topics that include the follow-up to the Warnock Report. He has previously worked in the Science and Engineering Research Council and the Department of Trade and Industry.

Sir Cecil Clothier, KCB, QC, Chairman of the Police Complaints Authority, was called to the Bar in 1950. He served as Parliamentary Commissioner for Administration, and Health Service Commissioner from 1979 to 1985 and was a member of the Royal Commission on the National Health Service from 1976 to 1985. He was a legal assessor to the General Medical Council and the General Dental Council from 1972 to 1978 and a member of the Merrison Committee on the regulation of the medical profession. He was Chairman of the Joint Committee of the medical and pharmaceutical professions to consider and report upon arrangements for dispensing in rural areas. He is a member of the MRC/RCOG Voluntary Licensing Authority for IVF and research.

Gordon Dunstan was ordained a priest in the Church of England in 1942. He is Emeritus Professor of Moral and Social Theology in the University of London, having been at King's College from 1967 to 1982. He is now Honorary Research Fellow at the University of Exeter and has been Chaplain to the Queen since 1976. He has served on the Advisory Groups on Transplant Policy and on Arms Control and Disarmament and on the Advisory Committee on Animal Experiments. He is a member of the MRC/RCOG Voluntary Licensing Authority for IVF and research. His publications include editions of mediaeval texts and analyses of contemporary ethical issues, including *The Artifice of Ethics* (1974), and, with A.S. Duncan and R.B. Welbourn, *A Dictionary of Medical Ethics* (2nd edn, 1981).

Anthony O. Dyson has been Samuel Ferguson Professor of Social and Pastoral Theology at the University of Manchester since 1980. After serving as Canon of St George's Chapel, Windsor Castle (1974–1977), he became Associate Director of the Centre for the Study of Religion and Society at Canterbury (1978–1980). He edited *The Teilhard Review* from 1966 to 1972 and has edited *The Modern Churchman* since 1982. He has published extensively on existentialism and theology.

Robert G. Edwards, FRS, is Professor of Human Embryology at the University of Cambridge and Scientific Director of Bourn Hall Clinic, Cambridge. His publications include *A Matter of Life* (with P.C. Steptoe, 1980), *Conception in the Human Female* (1980), and *Human Conception In Vitro* (with J.M. Purdy, 1982). He has edited several textbooks on reproduction and written numerous articles on this and related topics.

Antonia Gerard specialized in family law as a practitioner (at the Bar), as an academic (as Senior Lecturer, later Visiting Fellow, at the University of Southampton), and as judge (assistant recorder). Since 1982 she has been a conciliator attached to the Family Conciliation Bureau in Bromley,

Kent. Her published papers on various aspects of family law include 'Which mother: genetic or gestational?' (1983). She is now Legal Officer to the Foreign Compensation Commission.

Peter Harper is Professor of Medical Genetics at University of Wales College of Medicine, Cardiff, and Hospital of Wales. His main interests are in the field of genetic counselling and in the identification of the genes for major inherited neurological disorders. He is the author of *Myotonic Dystrophy* (1979), *Practical Genetic Counselling* (1984), and is editor of the *Journal of Medical Genetics*.

Geoffrey Hawthorn is a Reader in Sociology and Politics at Cambridge University. He has worked, among other things, on social aspects of fertility and on related policies both in Britain and in the Third World.

Michael Hull is Reader and Consultant in the University of Bristol Department of Obstetrics and Gynaecology. He is actively involved in clinical research and teaching on infertility. His publications cover the epidemiology of infertility, endocrinology of ovulation failure and induction, endometriosis, seminology, unexplained infertility, and *in vitro* fertilization, and he edited *Developments in Infertility Practice* (1981).

Teresa Iglesias, born in Salamanca, studied philosophy at Madrid University and University College, Dublin, where she was subsequently a lecturer. She obtained her doctorate from Oxford University and held a visiting fellowship at New Hall, Cambridge. She has written various papers on the philosophy of Wittgenstein and on ethics. Her most recent writings have been on the ethical issues raised by IVF and related techniques. She has been Research Officer at The Linacre Centre, a national Roman Catholic centre for the study of health care ethics, since 1981.

Howard Jacobs, Professor in the Department of Reproductive Endocrinology at the Middlesex Hospital School of Medicine, London, is an endocrinologist with a particular interest in reproduction. After training in general and laboratory endocrinology he worked in a department of obstetrics and gynaecology for eight years. At present his major interests are in the endocrine control of ovulation for *in vivo* and *in vitro* fertilization.

Martin H. Johnson is Reader in Experimental Embryology at Cambridge University and Fellow of Christ's College. He is currently Chairman of the British Society for Developmental Biology, and co-director, with Peter R. Braude, of an MRC-funded programme of research into early mouse and human development. He is co-author, with Barry J. Everitt, of *Essential Reproduction*, a teaching text on mammalian reproduction.

Stephen Lock has been editor of the *British Medical Journal* since 1975. Previously a haematologist, he was medical correspondent to the BBC Overseas Service from 1966 to 1974. He was appointed assistant editor of the *BMJ* in 1964, becoming deputy editor in 1974. Particularly interested in teaching medical writing, he has run many courses in Britain, Finland, Iraq, Kuwait, Canada, and Australia. He is a founder member of the International Committee of Medical Journal Editors and is immediate past president of the European Association of Science Editors. His books include *Thorne's Better Medical Writing*, *Family and Health Guide*, and *The Medical Risks of Life*.

Anne McLaren, FRS, is Director of the Medical Research Council's Mammalian Development Unit at University College London. She has worked on the reproductive and developmental biology of laboratory animals, including *in vitro* fertilization and embryo transfer, since the 1950s. She was a member of the DHSS Committee of Inquiry into

Human Fertilisation and Embryology chaired by Dame Mary Warnock, and at present chairs the Review Group of WHO's Human Reproduction Programme.

John Maddox, editor of *Nature* 1966–1973 and from 1980 onwards, was a lecturer on theoretical physics at Manchester University from 1949 to 1955 and was science correspondent of *The Guardian* from 1955 to 1964. He has served as a Member of the Royal Commission on Environmental Pollution, the UK Government Genetic Manipulation Advisory Group, the British Library Advisory Council, and Council on International Development.

Bernadette Modell is a Consultant and Wellcome Senior Lecturer in Perinatal Medicine at University College Hospital, London. She did her Ph.D. in developmental biology before studying medicine, and has subsequently concentrated on clinical research on all aspects of thalassaemia, taking this condition as an example of genetic disease. She has contributed to the development of management of the disease, and its prevention at the community level by carrier diagnosis, genetic counselling, and foetal diagnosis. Her unit is now a WHO Collaborative Centre for Community Control of the Haemoglobin-opathies.

Arthur Peacocke, born in 1924, is Director of the Ian Ramsey Centre, St Cross College, Oxford. For over 25 years he followed an academic career in the Universities of Birmingham and Oxford, working on the physical chemistry of biological macromolecules. His other chief interests have been in theology, the relation of science and theology, and philosophy of science. He was ordained as a priest in the Church of England in 1971 and was Dean of Clare College, Cambridge from 1973 to 1984. Recent publications include *Intimations of Reality; Critical Realism in Science and Religion* (1984) and *The Physical Chemistry of Biological Organization* (1983), and he has just edited a volume entitled *Reductionism in Academic Disciplines* (1985).

Charles H. Rodeck, born in 1944, is Senior Lecturer/Consultant in Obstetrics and Gynaecology and Director of the Harris Birthright Research Centre for Foetal Medicine in the Department of Obstetrics and Gynaecology, King's College School of Medicine and Dentistry, London.

David J. Weatherall, FRS, is Nuffield Professor of Clinical Medicine at the University of Oxford and Honorary Director of the MRC Molecular Haematology Unit. From 1971 to 1974 he was Professor of Haematology at the University of Liverpool. He has chaired several working parties for the World Health Organisation in work related to the abnormal haemoglobin disorders. His principal research interests are in the field of the thalassaemias and the regulation of haemoglobin synthesis during fetal development. His published work includes *The Thalassaemia Syndromes* (3rd edn, 1981).

Bernard Williams is Provost of King's College, Cambridge, having previously been Knightbridge Professor of Philosophy. He has written several books on moral philosophy, most recently *Ethics and the Limits of Philosophy* (1985).

Bob Williamson is Professor of Biochemistry at St Mary's Hospital Medical School, University of London. His research has focused on determining the causes of inherited disease through the use of cloned gene-specific probes. After cloning the globin genes and using them for the diagnosis of thalassaemia during the first trimester of pregnancy, he has studied Duchenne muscular dystrophy, cystic fibrosis, and coronary artery disease both by genetic linkage analysis and by studying candidate genes. He was a member of the UK Government Genetic Manipulation Advisory Group from its inception in 1976 until its demise in 1984, and has edited a series of books on genetic engineering.

Preface

The first child conceived with the help of *in vitro* fertilization techniques was born in July 1978. In the UK the legal and ethical issues raised by *in vitro* fertilization and by the research which makes IVF possible were later made the subject of a Committee of Inquiry set up by the Department of Health and Social Security and chaired by Dame Mary Warnock. The Warnock Committee's Report (1984) makes a number of specific recommendations, one of which is that research on human embryos should be permitted up to the fourteenth day after fertilization.

In February 1985 Mr Enoch Powell introduced in the House of Commons a Private Member's Bill that sought to prevent any experiments on human embryos. The Unborn Children (Protection) Bill would have made it an offence to create a human embryo, or to keep or use an embryo, for any purpose other than enabling a child to be born to a particular woman. It would also have made it an offence to be in possession of a human embryo without the explicit authority of the Secretary of State for Social Services. Neither this bill nor its successor has so far been passed by the House of Commons and although the government has stated that it intends to introduce legislation regulating embryo research, there are at present no such laws in the UK. In the interim the Medical Research Council has set up a Voluntary Licensing Authority to examine proposals for research on human embryos.

Since the Warnock Report was published there has been much public debate on the questions raised by human embryo research. These questions were the subject of a meeting held at the Ciba Foundation in November 1985 and recorded in this volume. The

Preface xv

study group focuses on the medical and scientific aspects of research on early human embryos but the contributors include representatives of the law, moral philosophy, and theology as well as science and medicine. We hope that the book will help to clarify the scientific issues for non-specialist readers and that it indicates where medical research could benefit from the use of early human embryos and where such research might not be justified.

Gregory Bock
Maeve O'Connor
March, 1986

ONE

Introduction: Research on early human embryos

Sir Cecil Clothier

As we get ever closer to knowing about that coalescence of organized particles which may be the beginning of another human being, the thrill of the chase, from the point of view of scientists, becomes greater and greater, and the anxiety of other people may increase in proportion. Every intelligent being must be curious about these matters, curiosity being one of the hallmarks of intelligence. For scientists there is always a strong incentive to press forward towards greater knowledge and greater control of any process, particularly this one. But at least half the human race needs, and frequently prefers, a mystery to precise knowledge of many matters. In particular the beginning of life, for a large proportion of the population, is a divine mystery which it may be profane to probe and expose too much. These two points of view are diametrically opposed and are properly entitled to mutual respect. We must recognize the virtual impossibility of one party being converted to the other.

One of the functions of law in society is to reconcile and control conflicting currents of human activity. Human activity is so diverse in its character that conflict is a more or less continuous state in society. The law provides a rough and ready basis, a very blunt instrument, with which to reconcile the conflicts that occur. One has to arrive at the lowest common denominator of acceptable conduct in any particular field of human endeavour which will enable people to live together and enable their inevitable disputes to be resolved with some sort of satisfaction.

One of the most useful functions of a study group such as this is to test opposed opinions about any matter in order to determine, if possible, the limits of acceptability of any particular form of activity. Here of course the activity is the one roughly described in the title, *Human Embryo Research*. This topic is complicated by the very strong emotions it arouses. These emotions are not confined to those who prefer mystery to science. Scientists too may have very strong emotions about their work and its validity and usefulness to humanity. They feel bitterly frustrated and angry if they are obstructed in what they see as the way forward to better and closer knowledge of the human organism and to ways of keeping it well and making it well to start with.

The emotional content of the topic probably arises from the instinctive and powerful respect that all decent people feel for the preservation of human life and the continuation of the species. Throughout history the law has shown a particular preoccupation with the sanctity of life. The law has provided for its protection from the earliest moment at which life could be perceived to have begun. Unfortunately the law follows behind both scientific knowledge and public opinion, sometimes a long way behind. It is therefore often unfitted and unable to deal with current problems. Even when it is designed for a current problem it tends to be a blunt instrument because it is incapable of dealing with every nuance and every subtlety of human relationship which may come under scrutiny.

It seems shocking to reflect that most of the many sections of the Offences Against the Person Act 1861 are still in force today. That was passed by Parliament at a time when phrases like 'quick with child' were still in common use. To decide whether a woman was pregnant you would enquire whether she was quick with child, meaning had there been movement of the foetus in the uterus. If not, perhaps life had not begun. There is a sort of logic about this but it is slightly shocking that we still have in force a law that only reflects our state of knowledge in 1861 of how and when life begins. This illustrates how far science has travelled while the law has almost stood still. The notion of protecting an embryo didn't enter the mind of the draftsman at that time.

Even in 1929, when protection to the child *in utero* was given by the Infant Life Preservation Act, it was given only to a child 'capable of being born alive'. The Act prescribed that evidence that the woman had been pregnant for twenty-eight weeks was *prima facie* proof that there was a child capable of being born alive. The scientists have been taking great leaps forward in understanding the mechanisms of reproduction, while the law has dragged lamentably behind and really does need overhauling as a matter of some urgency.

The ultimate and immensely difficult question is at what point coalescent and multiplying cells that are perhaps not even visible to the naked eye are entitled to our respect as a life in being and to all the care for its integrity and preservation which the law can provide. The attitude of our legislators to this difficult question is fraught with idiosyncrasy. An article in *The Times* for 31 October 1985 showed how deep the divisions on this subject are in Parliament and how widely they traverse the normal boundaries of party interest. Curious and uneasy partnerships and alliances may be formed. For example Mr Barney Hayhoe's support for Mr Enoch Powell's failed Bill is curious in political terms. [In the Unborn Children (Protection) Bill, February 1985, Mr Powell sought to ban all experiments on human embryos.]

Guidance on moral matters from our legislators is wavering and uncertain. One is reminded of the phenomenon known in the Admiralty Division of the High Court of Justice as a radar-assisted collision. The judgments made when the law is being interpreted are not much surer as aids to navigation. When Mrs Victoria Gillick challenged the right of doctors to prescribe contraceptives to girls under sixteen years of age without the consent of their parents, she lost by three to two in the House of Lords; but of the nine judges who considered the matter from start to finish, a majority (five) were in her favour. So where are we? That is another case more heavily charged with heat than light. It plainly behoves us to move with great caution as we approach the ultimate wonder of the commencement of human life, and also as we find that we can experiment and thus discover further facts about it. Those facts might include why the process sometimes begins well and results in a healthy and happy human being, and at other times results in quite the reverse.

There must be few who would dispute the benefits to

humankind of two major possibilities which may result from this area of research, that is to say, the cure and relief of infertility and the prevention of genetic disease. Indeed we might be willing to disregard the opinions of anyone who would dispute that those were potential benefits from this area of research. What is in question and a matter of anxiety is the process by which we research. It is those processes which are under attack where they involve, as it were, a seeming assault on a potential human life.

When I spoke earlier of the immensely difficult question of when a group of cells becomes entitled to our respect as a life in being, I only foreshadowed an even greater difficulty. Just as there are very few absolutes in philosophy, so there are few absolutes in physical and mental handicap. None of us can run or jump, physically or mentally, with precisely the same degree of agility. Who shall judge at what point our lack of abilities in either sphere is such that life is not even worth beginning, let alone continuing? That there is such a point I think is undeniable but defining it is almost impossible.

These are just some of the problems I have identified. In the uncreative way of lawyers, that is about all I am able to do. I cannot offer solutions but just point to where things get very difficult and then stand back and watch other people fight it out. This may however be the proper introductory task of the chairman in a gathering such as this. I am, after all, only a moderator of the proceedings and will listen with intense interest to what the experts in this field will tell us about the problems and difficulties that lie ahead.

TWO
Prelude to embryogenesis

A. McLaren

For most of its development, a mammalian oocyte (egg) is genetically similar to every other cell in the female's body. At the first meiotic division (triggered by a surge of luteinizing hormone – the 'LH surge') the oocyte becomes genetically unique, but neither its own genes nor the genes of the genetically unique sperm that fuses with it at fertilization start to function until after the first cleavage division. There ensues a period of totipotency, during which every cell of the pre-embryo is potentially capable of giving rise to every tissue in the adult body. Cell commitment begins at the mid-blastocyst stage and involves increasing numbers of cells during implantation, with groups separating off to form the trophoblast and other extra-embryonic tissues. The residual cells eventually form an embryonic plate on which may arise one or more primitive streaks, each giving rise to an individual embryo. This marks the onset of organogenesis, with each embryo developing into a foetus and then into a neonate.

Embryogenesis means 'the formation of the embryo' or 'the origin of the embryo'. But how far back should we look for origins? The continuous, cyclical nature of life has been emphasized by many authors (e.g. McLaren 1981). The great embryologist E.B. Wilson wrote in 1896 'Embryogenesis begins in oogenesis', so an appropriate point at which to begin the story of human embryogenesis is perhaps in the ovary, before fertilization, when the female germ cell (the oocyte or egg) resumes its development and becomes genetically unique.

Up to that point the oocyte has been genetically indistinguishable from millions of other cells in the woman's body and thousands of other oocytes in the same ovary. All these oocytes began their development as oocytes long before the woman herself was even born, but they came to a halt at about the time of her birth. Although they remained alive and metabolically active, they made no further progress until the onset of puberty. From then onwards, every month for the rest of the woman's reproductive lifetime, a group of oocytes started to grow.

Genetic uniqueness

At a certain stage in its growth, the oocyte becomes able to respond to a hormone signal, the luteinizing hormone (LH) surge, by completing the first meiotic division. This division reduces the number of chromosomes from 46 to 23, but − more important − only one of the two previously held copies of each gene is kept. It is this *random segregation* of the genetic material during meiosis that ensures that every oocyte is unique, genetically different now from the other cells in the body, and different from every other oocyte. The completion of the first meiotic division marks the end of the first phase of development (see Fig. 2.1).

During the second phase, fertilization takes place, restoring the chromosome number to 46 and joining the unique set of genes in the egg to the unique set in the sperm. But in the mouse, and probably in other mammals too, these genes are all 'silent': no gene expression takes place at this time. All the activity of the egg depends on substances manufactured earlier, under the control of the mother's genome. Most of the RNA that controls development in ovulated mouse eggs is made during the growth phase of the oocyte, one to three weeks before ovulation (Bachvarova and De Leon 1980), so it must be unusually stable. This material controls at least two developmental programmes: one triggered by the LH surge and another, still based on pre-existing genetic information,

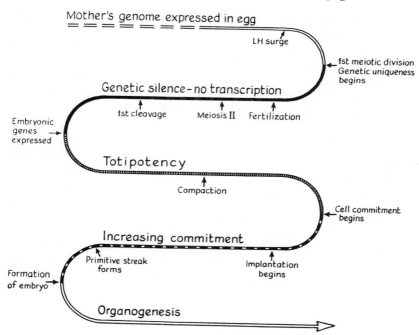

Mother's genome expressed in egg

LH surge

1st meiotic division
Genetic uniqueness
begins

Genetic silence - no transcription

1st cleavage   Meiosis II   Fertilization

Embryonic
genes →
expressed

Totipotency

Compaction

Cell commitment
begins

Increasing commitment

Primitive streak
forms

Implantation
begins

Formation
of embryo

Organogenesis

Figure 2.1 a generalized scheme to show the important stages of early mammalian development. During the first stage, which terminates at the time of the first meiotic division, the germ cells are genetically identical to other body cells of the parent. During the second, the germ cells and, after fertilization, the zygote are genetically unique but development is still controlled by the mother's genetic programme. During the third, the pre-embryo's own genes are expressed but the cells are not yet committed to any particular developmental fate. During the fourth, increasing numbers of cells are committed to extra-embryonic activities, providing the nutritive and protective life-support systems for the future embryo. During the fifth, an individual embryo can be recognized, in which tissue and organs develop. The diagram is not to scale: in the human, the first stage may last anything from ten to fifty years, the second about two days, the third about three days, the fourth eleven to twelve days, and the fifth about six weeks

triggered by fertilization (see Johnson, McConnell, and Van Blerkom 1984).

The human egg is normally shed from the ovary after the first meiotic division is completed but before fertilization [see Edwards, this volume, p. 40]. Egg maturation, the period between the completion of the first meiotic division and fertilization, is crucial if an embryo is later to develop normally. For *in vitro* fertilization (IVF) the egg must be recovered from the ovary before it is shed (Edwards 1980), so a greater or lesser part of the maturation period is spent *in vitro* in a culture system. For sheep eggs matured *in vitro* we know that the composition of the culture medium, in particular its hormone content, affects the pattern of protein synthesis in the egg; it also determines whether the egg can be fertilized and whether the fertilized egg is able to develop further (Moor and Trounson 1977; Moor, Polge, and Willadsen 1980). We do not yet have information of this kind for human egg maturation: perhaps some failures of IVF are due to inadequate conditions for maturation.

New gene set takes over

The period of genetic silence lasts through the events of egg maturation, fertilization, and the first cleavage division. It is ended, in the mouse, by a burst of transcription, that is synthesis of messenger RNA from DNA, during the two-cell stage (Bolton, Oades, and Johnson 1984). If this gene activity is inhibited by a drug, α-amanitin, the fertilized egg does not develop much further. The two-cell stage, an unusually long stage of cleavage in the mouse, also sees a massive breakdown of the maternal RNA, inherited in the egg cytoplasm. Evidently the new genome established at fertilization is now taking over control of development. This conclusion is strengthened by the expression at the two-cell stage (but not earlier) of genes known to have been transmitted from the father (see, e.g., Sawicki, Magnuson, and Epstein 1981).

The stage at which the new genome starts to function and so takes over control of development may vary from one mammalian species to another. So far the mouse is the only species for which we have accurate information. In the pig the switch may occur at the four-cell rather than the two-cell stage, as in this species it is the four-cell stage that is the longest cleavage stage. It will be important to collect information on gene expression during early human development, as this might enable genetic abnormalities to be recognized during cleavage *in vitro*; an unsuccessful pregnancy (or, worse, the birth of an abnormal baby) could then be avoided.

The burst of genetic activity at the two-cell stage causes a marked shift in the pattern of proteins synthesized in the mouse between the two- and four-cell stage. At the eight-cell stage a process termed compaction occurs (Johnson 1981): the cells flatten on one another and become wedge-shaped instead of spherical; at the same time they polarize, in such a way that their inner ends, in contact with other cells all round, show very different features from their outer ends. At the next cleavage most of these cells divide transversely, so the sixteen-cell stage consists of two rather different populations of cells – an inner and an outer. Shortly after this a fluid-filled cavity appears in the interior of the clump of cells: cleavage is completed and we now have a blastocyst, with an inner cell mass derived from the inner cells of the sixteen-cell stage and a peripheral layer of trophectoderm derived from the outer cells. The trophectoderm cells are important for implantation in the uterus and for the early nutrition of the embryo; some of these cells later form part of the foetal placenta.

Cell fate becomes restricted

Although two differentiated populations of cells, differing in both function and appearance, have emerged by the blastocyst stage, we know from experimental manipulations in the mouse that all these cells are totipotent. That is, if the cells are isolated or rearranged, each is capable of giving rise to both trophectoderm and inner cell mass. During cleavage the clump of cells derived from the fertilized egg can be split up to give rise to two blastocysts, or they can be aggregated with another such clump to give a single blastocyst, and development will still proceed normally. It is only at the mid-blastocyst stage that the cells become committed to their different fates, so trophectoderm cells can no longer give rise to inner cell mass, or inner cell mass to trophectoderm (Fleming *et al.* 1984).

In sheep and cattle, cleavage lasts longer than in mice and a much larger clump of cells is required before blastocyst formation begins. Cell commitment is correspondingly delayed. One consequence is that the clump can be divided into two or even four parts with little or no loss of developmental potential (Willadsen 1981; Willadsen *et al.* 1981). This procedure is now used commercially to increase the number of progeny developing from a single fertilized cow or sheep egg of high genetic worth. In the mouse, on the other hand, division of the cell clump into two (whether at the two-cell or sixteen-cell stage) greatly reduces the chances of successful development after implantation, while division into four parts has never yielded viable young. This is because the number of cells in the inner cell mass is reduced below the critical level required to give rise to an embryo later on. In terms of cell numbers and timing of blastocyst formation, early human development appears to resemble that in the mouse rather than that in sheep and cattle, but we have no direct evidence on when in human development cells are first committed to a particular future. The question is not entirely academic, as it has a bearing on how many cells could safely be removed for diagnosis of a genetic or chromosomal defect without jeopardizing subsequent development (McLaren 1984).

Implantation

We have now reached the end of the third phase of development as outlined in Fig. 2.1. From the mid-blastocyst stage onwards, over the implantation period, more and more cells become committed to form the various tissues and structures collectively known as extra-embryonic membranes, concerned with the process of implantation and with the protection and nutrition of the future embryo, while the domain of relatively uncommitted cells becomes a progressively smaller and smaller part of the whole.

Implantation in women takes about a week, from about six to thirteen days after fertilization. During this time the trophoblast (derived from the outer trophectoderm layer of the blastocyst) becomes firmly anchored within the wall of the uterus and little fingers (chorionic villi) of a different population of trophectoderm cells push into the maternal blood spaces to absorb nutrients. After the trophectoderm has differentiated, the next cell population to become committed is the primary endoderm. This forms the inner lining of the yolk sac which is thought to contribute to the nutrition of the implanting blastocyst. The relatively uncommitted residue of the inner cell mass, now termed the epiblast, forms the upper layer, one cell thick, of the small central embryonic plate. The amniotic cavity develops as a split between the epiblast and the adjacent trophoblast (Luckett 1975). The extra-embryonic mesoblast, at one time thought to arise from the trophectoderm, now seems more likely to come from a proliferating region at one end of the epiblast (Luckett 1978). The mesoblast surrounds the yolk sac and amniotic cavity and also forms a central core to each chorionic villus, contributing largely to the foetal placenta.

Once implantation has been completed, the only cells not committed to an extra-embryonic fate are a group of a few thousand in the epiblast layer of the embryonic plate. It is in the embryonic plate that the primitive streak is formed, with the epiblast cells piling up to make a groove through which they move to give rise to a third layer of cells in the interior of the embryonic plate. Usually a single primitive streak develops, marking the position of the embryo and then of the foetus. Sometimes no streak appears (perhaps because the embryonic plate contains too few cells), in which case no embryo develops and the pregnancy ends (the 'blighted ovum'). Sometimes two primitive streaks form and monozygotic twins develop, sharing a single amnion and placenta. The primitive streak stage is the latest stage at which twinning can take place, marking the onset of individual embryonic development.

An embryo at last

The last extra-embryonic tissue to be split off from the epiblast is the allantois, which in human development combines with the extra-embryonic mesoblast to form the umbilical cord. By this time, about sixteen days after fertilization, all the cells derived from the fertilized egg are finally committed to being either part of the individual embryo or outside it. Since we now have a spatially defined entity that can develop directly into a foetus and thence into a baby, we are for the first time justified in using the term 'embryo'. This entity has often been referred to by embryologists as the 'definitive embryo' or 'the embryo proper', the term 'embryo' being reserved either for the early stages before any extra-embryonic tissues have differentiated or for the totality of cells derived from the fertilized egg. This usage understandably leads to confusion. In lower animals, from which most embryological terminology derives, the ambiguity does not arise since there are no extra-embryonic tissues. For mammals it seems preferable to use the term 'pre-embryo' or 'conceptus' for the entire product of the fertilized egg up to the end of the implantation stage (some fourteen days after ovulation in humans), and 'embryo' for that small part of the pre-embryo or conceptus, first distinguishable at the primitive streak stage, that later develops into the foetus.

Up to about 18 days after ovulation (Carnegie stage 7: see Table 2.1), the embryo is still less than a millimetre in length (Fig. 2.2) and contains no differentiated tissue or organs. Its genetic constitution is usually the same as that of the fertilized egg, but in rare cases a chromosome may be lost or gained or modified during the intervening couple of weeks. With monozygotic twinning, this may lead to the surprising result of so-called 'identical' twins of opposite sex. Published reports of discordant monozygotic twins are summarized in a recent account of a set of monozygotic triplets consisting of two boys with a normal XY chromosome complement and a girl with an XO chromosome complement, expressed in Turner's syndrome (Dallapiccola *et al.* 1985).

In the final phase of development included in Fig. 2.1, the embryo embarks on organogenesis. This process again consists of the successive commitment of groups of cells, but now it is the commitment of groups of cells within the embryo, to form different tissues and organs. The first sign of organ formation is the closure of the neural folds to form the neural tube at the beginning of the fourth week of development. The neural tube folds and bulges to form the brain vesicles, the cranial nerves begin to grow out at about five weeks, and the first morphological indications of a cerebral cortex can be seen by about six weeks.

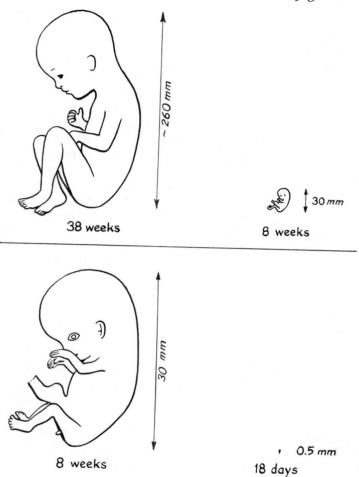

Figure 2.2   the relative size of a baby at birth, a foetus at the beginning of the foetal stage, and an embryo near the start of embryonic development (after Moore 1977). The upper two drawings are about a quarter life size, the lower two about twice life size

Eight weeks (Table 2.1) marks the beginning of the foetal period, the stage when all the main structures of the body have been formed. Function in the nervous system becomes established gradually, during the foetal period and after birth.

At this meeting we shall be mainly concerned with the first two weeks of human development, the 'pre-embryonic' stage. Many (perhaps most) fertilized eggs fail to survive this stage, so it is evident that its successful accomplishment is not easy, but it is crucial for all subsequent development. This stage is essentially a period of preparation, during which all the protective and nutritive systems required for the support of the future embryo are elaborated. Once the support systems are established the embryo itself, as an individual entity, can begin to develop.

The Ciba Foundation has organized two previous symposia on early development. The timing of those meetings was significant. The first, on *Preimplantation Stages of Pregnancy* in 1965, was held towards the end of the pioneering period of studies of mammalian development, when *in vitro* culture and manipulations such as the production of aggregation chimeras were new and exciting. The terms 'embryo' and 'ovum' were at that time used interchangeably. The decade that followed saw an explosive rise in research on preimplantation stages in mice. In 1975 the time seemed ripe to push forward into the technically more demanding and conceptually more complex postimplantation period, so the symposium on *Embryogenesis in Mammals* made an attempt, only partially successful, to focus attention on postimplantation development. My own enthusiasm for those two symposia was based partly on a feeling that they would benefit the discipline of embryology, but also, I confess, on a strong desire to reduce my own ignorance of what seemed important and exciting areas of knowledge. Indeed, it was while I was trying to put together for the 1975 symposium a growth curve for the whole of mouse prenatal development that it first began to dawn on me that the 'embryo' as a continuous entity could be traced back from birth only as far as the primitive streak stage (six days after fertilization in mice), and that the 'embryo' that develops from fertilization onwards is a different entity, which includes and gives rise to the 'embryo' that grows into a foetus and neonate but is in no way coextensive with it. It has taken a further ten years and some

Table 2.1 The timing of early human development[a]

	time relative to ovulation (days)	Carnegie stage[b]
LH[c] surge begins	$-1\frac{1}{2}$	
ovulation	0	
fertilization	$\frac{1}{2}-1\frac{1}{2}$	1
two to sixteen cells	2–4	2
blastocyst	5	3
trophectoderm differentiates	4–6	
implantation begins	6–7	4
primary endoderm differentiates	6–7	
amniotic cavity formed	8	
trophoblast proliferates	7–12	5
extra-embryonic mesoblast develops	8–13	
implantation complete	13–14	
chorionic villi form	13–15	6
primitive streak develops	15–18	
allantois forms	16–18	7
neural tube begins to close	22–23	10
first sign of cerebral cortex	42	17
foetal stage begins	56	23

[a]Different authorities may differ by a day or two in the times that they give for various developmental events. In part this is due to problems of definition (e.g. when does 'implantation' begin and end?), but in part it reflects biological variation and our lack of precise knowledge of early human development. The times given in this table are taken from O'Rahilly (1973) and from Moore (1977).
[b]The Carnegie stages were proposed by O'Rahilly (1973); although arbitrary, they are useful for purposes of comparison.
[c]LH, luteinizing hormone.

pressure from outside the scientific community for this distinction to result in a suggested change of terminology to eliminate the ambiguity of the term 'embryo'.

References

Bachvarova, R. and De Leon, V. (1980) Polyadenylated RNA of mouse ova and loss of maternal RNA in early development. *Developmental Biology* 74: 1–8

Bolton, V.N., Oades, P.J., and Johnson, M.H. (1984) The relationship between cleavage, DNA replication, and gene expression in the mouse 2-cell embryo. *Journal of Embryology and Experimental Morphology* 79: 139–63

Ciba Foundation (1965) *Preimplantation Stages of Pregnancy*. London: J. & A. Churchill (Ciba Foundation Symposium) 442 pp.

Ciba Foundation (1976) *Embryogenesis in Mammals*. Amsterdam: Elsevier (Ciba Foundation Symposium 40) 316 pp.

Dallapiccola, B., Stomeo, C., Ferranti, G., Di Lecce, A., and Purpura, M. (1985) Discordant sex in one of three monozygotic triplets. *Journal of Medical Genetics* 22: 6–11

Edwards, R.G. (1980) *Conception in the Human Female*. London: Academic Press

Fleming, T.P., Warren, P.D., Chisholm, J.C., and Johnson, M.H. (1984) Trophectodermal processes regulate the expression of totipotency within the inner cell mass of the mouse expanding blastocyst. *Journal of Embryology and Experimental Morphology* 84: 63–90

Johnson, M.H. (1981) The molecular and cellular basis of preimplantation mouse development. *Biological Reviews* 56: 463–98

Johnson, M.H., McConnell, J., and Van Blerkom, J. (1984) Programmed development in the mouse embryo. *Journal of Embryology and Experimental Morphology* 83 (Supplement): 197–231

Luckett, W.P. (1975) The development of primordial and definitive amniotic cavities in early rhesus monkey and human embryos. *American Journal of Anatomy* 144: 149–67

Luckett, W.P. (1978) Origin and differentiation of the yolk sac and extraembryonic mesoderm in presomite human and rhesus monkey embryos. *American Journal of Anatomy* 152: 59–97

McLaren, A. (1981) *Germ Cell and Soma: A New Look at an Old Problem*. New Haven and London: Yale University Press

McLaren, A. (1984) Prenatal diagnosis before implantation: opportunities and problems. *Prenatal Diagnosis* 5: 85–90

Moor, R.M. and Trounson, A.O. (1977) Hormonal and follicular factors affecting maturation of sheep oocytes *in vitro* and their subsequent developmental capacity. *Journal of Reproduction and Fertility* 49: 101–109

Moor, R.M., Polge, C., and Willadsen, S.M. (1980) Effect of follicular steroids on the maturation and fertilization of mammalian oocytes. *Journal of Embryology and Experimental Morphology* 56: 319–35

Moore, K.L. (1977) *The Developing Human*, 2nd edn. Philadelphia: Saunders

O'Rahilly, R. (1973) *Development Stages in Human Embryos, Part A:*

Embryos of the First Three Weeks (Stages 1–9). Carnegie Institute of Washington, Washington DC (Publication 631)

Sawicki, W., Magnuson, T., and Epstein, C. (1981) Evidence for expression of the paternal genome in the two-cell mouse embryo. *Nature* 294: 450–54

Willadsen, S.M. (1981) The developmental capacity of blastomeres from 4-cell and 8-cell sheep embryos. *Journal of Embryology and Experimental Morphology* 65: 165–72

Willadsen, S.M., Lehn-Jensen, H., Fehilly, C.B., and Newcomb, R. (1981) The production of monozygotic twins of preselected parentage by micromanipulation of non-surgically collected cow embryos. *Theriogenology* 15: 23–9

Discussion

Clothier: Each of the stages you described is essential to the next. Each is a cause of the following effect. So which one do you choose as the initiating cause of human life?

McLaren: I don't think one can say when human life begins. The life process is continuous and for the very beginning one has to go back thousands of millions of years. I see development as a series of bottlenecks or discontinuities, as in the diagram (Fig. 2.3).

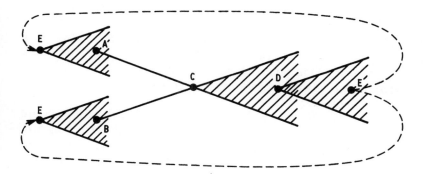

Figure 2.3   development as a series of discontinuous events. A, B: parental germ cells; C: fertilization; D: cells from which the embryo develops; E: primordial germ cells

Since one has to start somewhere, we may start with the germ cells (A and B in Fig. 2.3) that come together at fertilization (C). Each of these germs cells has arisen in the course of development of the germ cell population in the gonad of one of the parents. One can pick out that particular cell and retrospectively say where it started off as a genetically unique cell. From the fertilized egg a population of cells grows and develops. Then from this population a subset of cells (D) arises from which the embryo develops. A third such point is the origin of the primordial germ cells (E) during embryonic development. These cells arise as a subset of the population of embryo cells, again as a discontinuity. There is a sense in which these bottlenecks are discontinuities in a continuous process. I don't know whether that makes it any easier to think about but we can't say that life begins at any particular time.

Modell: In early development and fertilization great care is taken to arrange meiosis so that the chromosomes and genes get thoroughly mixed up, and each gamete is ultimately unique. This coincides with a tremendous superabundance of gametes and, in some species, also of individuals. Many species produce huge numbers of fertilized embryos which tend to get reduced until the species is just reproducing itself. In humans a similar reduction seems to happen very early after fertilization, at around the time of implantation and early embryonic development. In many other species it happens much later. That seems to be a key issue.

Williamson: How many pre-embryos are spontaneously aborted?

Modell: For the very early stages of pregnancy there is a certain amount of disagreement still. The fertilized ovum produces gonadotropin to prepare the uterus for implantation, and this can be measured in the mother's blood in the first few weeks of pregnancy. Such measurements indicate that about 60 per cent of fertilized ova fail to become implanted, and so cannot develop further. At seven or eight weeks of pregnancy ultrasound shows, with more certainty, that about 15 per cent of pregnancies where the ovum has become implanted are non-viable. These then progress to a spontaneous abortion. It also appears that in about 10 per cent of all pregnancies there are two gestation sacs. In 90 per cent of these, one of the twin sacs does not produce a living embryo, because the birth frequency of twins is only 1 per cent. There are a lot of very fascinating processes in the early stages of pregnancy.

Williamson: So a best estimate might be that between two-thirds and three-quarters of fertilizations spontaneously abort?

Modell: Yes; or the fertilized ova don't implant.

Clothier: The implication is that because nature is careless of fertilized ova they are less entitled to respect. In one discussion I heard it was argued that because nature herself was prodigal and tended to reject large numbers of eggs, experiments on surplus eggs were justified. I am not sure how that argument ought to proceed.

Modell: There is no justification for considering any living thing with a lack of respect. A superabundance is created at one point, after the careful sorting out of the genes and their rearrangement in new combinations. The subsequent natural reduction of this abundance doesn't imply any lack of respect but is a selection process whereby some fertilized ova are chosen as more viable than others. We don't understand the mechanisms yet. If we consider ourselves as part of nature, it might be reasonable to consider research as treating the eggs with respect, and to view selections made by us as part of the natural selection process.

Dunstan: I very much agree with that reply. I don't believe in the argument that because nature is wasteful we may be prodigal. I believe that scientific intervention at this point is precisely to increase selectivity in an evolutionary process in which what to us is waste is in fact a selection for biological, evolutionary ends. We are, in a way, aligned with a selective force against what appears to be an otherwise wasteful use of material.

Peacocke: Selection at this stage concerns the viability of the cell with respect to the next stage in the process of implantation and growth. Whether or not selection occurs with respect to the genetic constitution involved in other qualities, such as intelligence, that are important later in life, is problematic. We must be careful not to equate what is being selected for at this early stage with what is later advantageous to the whole organism in its environment as an adult.

Modell: Embryos are selected for their ability to survive in the environment they are in at any given stage. This process of selection is continuous throughout pregnancy as different genes are switched on to maintain the embryo at different stages of pregnancy. There is a progressive selection which is much more intensive earlier on and gradually becomes more subtle later.

Peacocke: Yes, there is a selection in response to the same conditions as appear later on. It is necessary that the fertilized cell survive this early stage, but other factors must operate later.

Williamson: A very high proportion of the genes of the embryo are switched on very early, much more than at later stages. If anything, molecular biology data would argue that selection could operate very early on expressed genes.

Edwards: We do not yet know if the embryos that survive are more likely to cleave more rapidly or activate their genes more quickly. The whole thing is wide open. I do not accept that embryonic loss is as high as 60 per cent just after implantation. That conclusion is based on the transitory secretion of human chorionic gonadotropin in plasma by the embryo dying early, but there are a lot of questions about the data. This type of embryonic loss would be expected after *in vitro* fertilization, but it is found only rarely.

Iglesias: First I should like to make a comment on the opening words of Sir Cecil Clothier. I come from a background of professional philosophy where the philosophical attitude is recognized to begin in wonder about the mysteries of existence and of the ultimate meaning and value of human life. Scientists, however, by their scientific attitude and investigations seek precise knowledge about that dimension of reality which is unknown or 'mysterious'; yet it is a dimension that can become known by methods of observation and experimentation. But not all dimensions of reality are amenable to the scientific eye. The value of human life and existence cannot be ascertained by looking at it under the microscope, nor can it be accounted for in terms of molecules. The philosophical and scientific attitudes are not incompatible but complementary and jointly necessary to the understanding of the individual person. Einstein is a good example of harmonizing these two attitudes. In his investigations he never lost his openness towards the mysteries of human life and existence. We may know *how* things exist and function, but *why* are they there at all? Why do I exist? Why a *being* rather than *nothing*?

A second point. The scientific account of life as cyclical does not preclude a philosopher, or the ordinary person, from wondering about his or her beginnings. Is it not a legitimate question to ask the scientists: when did I begin as a living organism or as a bodily being? Everyone understands that life considered in terms of cells with molecules and genes goes back millions and millions of years. But our everyday perceptions raise a legitimate question: when did I begin as a bodily being? Perhaps scientists need to enter a different framework of understanding and to regard organic entities as *whole living beings*, not merely as collections of molecules or cells. Houses may be viewed as collections of bricks that can be put up step by step and dismantled, as clocks can. But this is not so with the living being. The living being is generated as a whole, grows as a whole, and dies as a whole. We need more opportunities like this gathering for scientists and philosophers to discuss our understanding of life.

McLaren: Since your question is a semiphilosophical one, there are going to be many different answers. My answer comes directly from my crude diagram of discontinuities (Fig.

2.3). If we are talking not about the origin of life, as our Chairman said, but about the origin of an individual life, one can trace back directly from the newborn baby to the foetus, and back further to the origin of the individual embryo at the primitive streak stage in the embryonic plate at sixteen or seventeen days. If one tries to trace back further than that there is no longer a coherent entity. Instead there is a larger collection of cells, some of which are going to take part in the subsequent development of the embryo and some of which aren't. In most cases one can trace the genetic constitution back from the origin of the embryo, right to fertilization. But there are rare cases where a genetic accident happens between fertilization and the primitive streak stage, such that a chromosome is lost or gained. That is why, for instance, there are monozygotic twins (so-called 'identical' twins) in which one twin is a boy and the other is a girl who has lost the Y chromosome. Normally, though, you can trace the genetic constitution back all the way to fertilization. You can then trace back the genetic constitution of each gamete to where the oocyte and the sperm first arose as genetically unique cells within the mass of germ cells in the parents' gonads. You can't trace the genetic constitution back further than the completion of meiosis because that gene set would no longer be a discrete gene set but would be muddled up with all the other genes in the larger gene set of the parent. To me the point at which I began as a total whole individual human being was at the primitive streak stage, the formation of the embryo, but if one took a genetic viewpoint one could go back either to fertilization or to the two meiotic events occurring in the parents' gonads before fertilization.

Iglesias: I am grateful for this genetic view, but the philosopher would say that what constitutes a unique human is not merely that person's genes but his or her organic wholeness and subjectivity. This is recognized by experience, i.e. the experience of being a person who has a history of individual organic development which began before one was conscious of it. Many people recognize that the human being, like any other living being, begins as a whole and grows as a whole.

Clothier: We have now seen that a life can be traced back either to a cellular entity or to a genetic entity. Which of those is the valid view? One can only go back to a certain stage of a cellular clump and say 'That is me' but genetically one can go further back and still pick up a trail of ancestry.

Modell: For clarity Anne McLaren chose to go backwards in time, starting with a specific individual and going back to the gametes: but if you were to try to go forward in time, i.e. start with given gametes and move forward to an individual, you wouldn't be able to do the same thing, because in most cases there would be no final individual, in any sense that we understand. In processes with such a strong 'historical' component the 'arrow of time' is unidirectional. I find this a most interesting philosophical point.

THREE

Infertility: Nature and extent of the problem

M.G.R. Hull

The investigation and treatment of infertility has been studied in a group of 708 couples residing in a single administrative health district in England. The annual attendance rate of couples at specialist clinics was 472, representing 1.2 couples per 1000 of the total population in the district. It appears that at least one in six couples need specialist help at some time in their lives because of infertility that has lasted for an average of two and a half years; 71 per cent of those needing help are trying for their first baby. Ovulation failure (amenorrhoea, oligomenorrhoea) occurred in 21 per cent of women and was very successfully treated (two-year conception rates 96 per cent, 78 per cent). Tubal damage (14 per cent of women) had a poor outlook, with only about 19 per cent conceiving, despite surgery. Endometriosis accounted for infertility in 6 per cent (although seldom by tubal damage), cervical mucus defects or dysfunction in 3 per cent, and coital failure in up to 6 per cent. Sperm defects or dysfunction were the commonest defined cause of infertility (24 per cent) and led to a poor chance of pregnancy (0–27 per cent) when donor insemination was not used for treatment. Obstructive azoospermia and primary spermatogenic failure were uncommon (2 per cent) and hormonal causes of male infertility were rare. Infertility was unexplained in 28 per cent of couples and the chance of pregnancy (overall 72 per cent) was mainly determined by the duration of infertility. In vitro fertilization could benefit 80 per cent of women with tubal damage and 25 per cent of couples with unexplained infertility, i.e. 18 per cent of all infertile couples, representing up to 216 new couples each year per million total population.

Most people have a deep instinctive desire for children of their own, to love and be loved by them. Most people who have children (whom they don't always see as a blessing!) cannot imagine the transformation and emptiness of their lives if they had failed to have children. Infertility leads to deep and desperate longing that can overshadow everything else. It blights whole lives and sometimes leads to suicide. The grief is usually kept private, however, and the infertile are unwilling campaigners. Their problem is commonly seen as trivial, yet they deserve medical help as much as anyone else. They certainly deserve as much help as the fertile, for whom everything is provided: contraception, sterilization, abortion.

In this chapter I am primarily concerned, however, not with the emotional nature of infertility but with its physical nature, that is with the range of causes of infertility and with the effectiveness of treatment. This study then leads to an assessment of the newer medical resources needed. I am concerned with determining these needs in a way that would apply throughout the UK (and similar countries), as the focus is on a true population, resident in a particular area; in other words the results should be free of the usual bias that arises when infertility statistics are reported from research clinics with specialized interests. The Warnock Report (1984) drew attention to the lack of population statistics on infertility. The information I will give appears to be the first aimed at filling this gap. It is derived from a recent study reported in detail elsewhere (Hull *et al.* 1985).

The overpopulation of the world with people is due not to their efficient reproduction but to their efficient survival. Human fertility is poor compared with that of most domestic and laboratory animals. The peak conception rate in populations of proven fertility is only about 33 per cent in each ovulation cycle; the average is only about 20 per cent. Only 90 per cent of *fertile* couples conceive in their first year of trying, and 95 per cent in two years (Tietze 1956, 1968). In general, female fertility seems remarkably dependable and predictable, the main risk being from infective damage to the Fallopian tubes. The chance of conception is probably determined mainly by male fertility. Human sperm quality is relatively poor in general and when it is defined as abnormal it is at present virtually untreatable.

It is essential to understand the chance nature of fertility. It is never absolute; it can never be guaranteed. That is, it is never 100 per cent – not until *after* the event! Like the roll of a dice, there is no guarantee that everyone will eventually throw a six. The apparent slowing in the rate at which the chance of conception accumulates with the passage of time (as demonstrated later in Fig. 3.3) is in fact to be expected by the laws of chance. On the other hand, while fertility is never absolute, infertility is also rarely absolute, that is with zero chance of conception. Absolute infertility occurs, for instance, due to a premature menopause, or complete obstruction of both Fallopian tubes, or damage to the testicles causing complete lack of sperms (azoospermia). In practice, the usual need is for the lowered chance of conception – that is, the degree of subfertility, rather than true infertility – to be assessed accurately so that 'infertile' couples can decide whether their hope of conceiving with or without treatment is good or unrealistically low, and therefore what to do about it.

The definition of 'infertility' thus depends on its duration. Failure to conceive after a year is taken to be abnormal, as 90 per cent of fertile couples succeed within that time. Of course there are exceptions when help seems appropriate sooner, but the report that follows only applies to couples with at least one year's infertility. Permanent infertility may be infrequent but that is of remote interest in practice to couples who want a child. There are also some women who conceive but miscarry and others with a child who may find themselves unable to conceive again; these must also be taken into account.

Incidence and causes of infertility in the population

My study (Hull *et al.* 1985) describes infertility in a defined population (393000 at the time of study) in one of the three administrative health districts in and around Bristol (the Bristol and Weston Health District). It does not describe the complete picture of infertility, either in the whole resident population or to any fixed point in time. It describes a minimum picture, expressed by the annual attendance of new couples at specialist clinics, after couples from other districts have been excluded. In every case infertility lasted at least one year; on average it lasted two and a half years.

Incidence

The study focuses on new couples who first attended a clinic during part of 1982 and 1983. The annual rate of new couples attending was 472, which represents 1.2 couples a year per 1000 people in the general population. The study indicates that one in six couples (17 per cent) require specialist help for infertility at some time in their lives, with one in eight couples (13 per cent) needing help for a first child (previous pregnancy rates are discussed later).

The following findings are based on detailed information on 708 couples attending my own clinic during part of 1982 and 1983. Most (78 per cent) of the local couples are seen here and the findings are therefore taken to be representative. The average age of the women was twenty-eight years, whether they were trying for the first or for a subsequent pregnancy. The women were only eighteen months older than fertile women on average, when they started trying for their first pregnancy, suggesting that most infertility is unrelated to postponing attempts to conceive. The average age of the men was thirty-one years.

Causes

The distribution of causes of infertility is summarized in Fig. 3.1. Details of the investigations on which the classification is based are discussed in the original report (Hull *et al.* 1985), but in summary the investigations are: (1) menstrual history; (2) laparoscopy (using a narrow telescope to look inside the woman's abdomen under anaesthetic, enabling the best assessment of the pelvic organs, including the Fallopian tubes); (3) testing penetration of cervical mucus by sperms, generally after natural intercourse (the postcoital test), and if necessary using separate mucus and semen samples in the laboratory, including samples from normal donors (the crossed penetration test); (4) coital

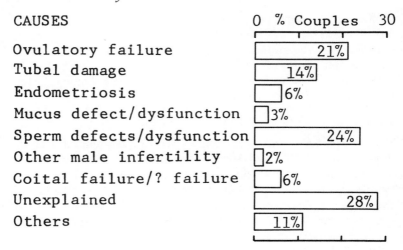

CAUSES   0 % Couples 30

Ovulatory failure   21%
Tubal damage   14%
Endometriosis   6%
Mucus defect/dysfunction   3%
Sperm defects/dysfunction   24%
Other male infertility   2%
Coital failure/? failure   6%
Unexplained   28%
Others   11%

Figure 3.1 percentage frequency distribution of causes found for infertility in a representative population of 708 couples defined by residence in a single administrative health district. (The total amounts to more than 100 per cent because 15 per cent of couples had two or more causes.)

history. Additional routine testing of secondary importance includes measurement of the levels of progesterone to assess ovulation, and seminal analysis.

The primary indication of sperm dysfunction is the inability of sperms to penetrate normal mucus. Given this finding, seminal analysis is used only to distinguish between men with obvious sperm defects and others with apparently normal semen classified as dysfunctional (see Fig. 3.1). The dysfunction evidenced by failure of mucus penetration is associated with impaired fertilizing ability that can be shown in the laboratory (*in vitro*) with both human (Wardle *et al.* 1985) and hamster eggs (Schats *et al.* 1984). Men with reduced sperm counts (oligospermia) but normal mucus penetration have demonstrably normal fertility (Glazener *et al.* 1985) and are therefore treated by me as normal.

I have dwelt on the diagnosis of sperm defects and dysfunction because they are the commonest defined cause of infertility (Fig.

3.1) but diagnostic inaccuracy remains a fundamental problem that undermines both practice and research in male infertility. It is misleading to assume that all men with low sperm counts are infertile, and equally that those with normal counts are fertile. Indeed it is also usually wrong to assume that sperm–mucus penetration failure is due to mucus 'hostility'. Sperm penetration of normal mucus is the simplest indirect index of the essential function of sperms: their fertilizing ability. That is the criterion applied in the classification shown in Fig. 3.1, and it is validated by its power in predicting pregnancy, as demonstrated later in Fig. 3.3.

In Fig. 3.1, ovulatory failure is defined as the absence of menstrual periods (amenorrhea) or as infrequent periods (oligomenorrhoea). Deficiency in the luteal phase of the cycle occurs in women with normal menstrual cycles but this condition is ignored because it is uncertain whether it occurs persistently enough to contribute to prolonged infertility. Cervical mucus defects (implying inherent inability to produce apparently normal preovulatory mucus) and dysfunction (normal-looking mucus that is unreceptive to normal sperms) are very uncommon. Sperm defects and dysfunction, already defined, represent the commonest defined abnormality accounting for infertility. 'Other male infertility' implies complete absence of sperms, whether due to obstruction of ducts, to testicular damage causing permanent inability to produce sperms, or to hypogonadotropism (a rare hormonal condition that is the only cause of male infertility which is reliably treatable). Coital 'failure' implies mainly infrequency of sexual intercourse; '? failure' implies that a problem is suspected because normal sperm–mucus penetration is found *in vitro* after negative postcoital tests. 'Unexplained infertility' is the biggest class, defined by normal findings in the complete set of basic investigations. Whether there is a real abnormality in such cases will be discussed later. Finally, there remains a group of 'others' which includes a few rare causes but consists mainly of couples who did not complete the investigations, some of whom conceived. The sum of all the diagnostic groups amounts to more than 100 per cent because two or more causes of infertility were found in 15 per cent of couples.

Previous pregnancy

Previous pregnancy rates are shown in Fig. 3.2, related to the cause of present infertility. Overall, 41 per cent of women had been pregnant (i.e. were parous), including 11 per cent who had had a therapeutic termination of pregnancy (TOP); 29 per cent had had a child, i.e. a pregnancy lasting at least twenty-eight weeks, although not always surviving. There were parous women in every diagnostic group. However, previous pregnancy appeared to contribute significantly to tubal damage causing infertility; the proportion of women with tubal damage who had had a child was 1.5 times the average, and the proportion who had had a previous termination was twice the average. A previous termination was also twice as likely in couples with coital problems, possibly reflecting original or consequent psychological problems. Couples with unexplained infertility were more likely (1.4 times the average) to have had a child, possibly

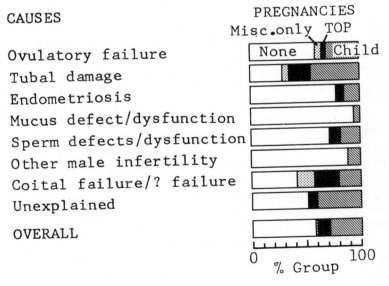

Figure 3.2 percentage of infertile women in each diagnostic group who had had a previous pregnancy. Misc.: miscarriage; TOP: therapeutic termination of pregnancy

reflecting the essentially chance nature of their infertility in the majority (see later). A previous pregnancy was relatively uncommon in women with endometriosis or mucus defects, or whose husbands had clearly defined sperm defects, suggesting a persisting inherent condition.

Effectiveness of treatment and future needs

The results of treatment in the main diagnostic groups are shown in Fig. 3.3, which refers to 584 couples with a single cause of infertility or with unexplained infertility, compared with normal. Only single causes have been studied, in order to allow the true effectiveness of treatment to be assessed.

The most successful treatment is for women with ovulatory failure, especially with amenorrhoea. The less successful results in women with oligomenorrhoea are mainly due to polycystic ovary disease, which is the only problem with no reliable solution. Tubal damage (excluding operative sterilization, not included here) is a major problem both because of its frequency and the very poor chance that surgery will be effective (treatment by *in vitro* fertilization [IVF] is not included in Fig. 3.3). The effectiveness of surgery is limited by irreversible infective damage to the tubal lining and fimbriae. Allowing for surgery, the only hope for 80 per cent of women with tubal damage would be by IVF.

In male infertility the outlook for a couple is poor unless artificial insemination by a donor (AID) is used; this is not included in the results in Fig. 3.3 because it is not a true cure for the problem but only bypasses it. There is no treatment of proven value in improving sperm function in infertile men, and artificial insemination by the husband (AIH) is of no benefit (as found in an as yet unpublished study in my clinic). IVF has generally been found disappointing but may prove useful as the ultimate test of male fertility.

The need for AID would apply to at least 80 per cent of cases of male infertility. Only a minority accept it at present but it will be taken up increasingly, firstly as diagnostic accuracy improves, particularly in men with seemingly normal 'sperm counts', and secondly as it becomes more generally understood that male

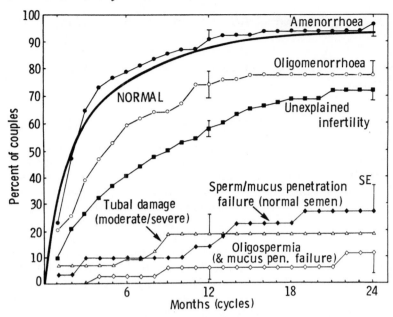

Figure 3.3 cumulative conception rates in 584 couples with a single cause of infertility, treated as appropriate, compared with normal rates (that is, with the highest rates reported in couples of proven fertility: Tietze 1956; 1968). The use of AID or IVF is excluded from these results. Unexplained infertility was untreated. SE: standard error of proportions, which is an index of the confidence limits for the conception rates shown. (Based on Hull *et al.* 1985.)

fertility has nothing to do with potency and the sense of shame is lost.

The results for unexplained infertility in Fig. 3.3 apply to couples who received no treatment. The group is heterogeneous. This is not the place to discuss all the possible causes that have been suggested, but it is at least clear that inclusion of laparoscopyand postcoital testing goes a long way to excluding previously unsuspected major causes. The unexplained group is the one group in which the duration of infertility (and to a much lesser extent the woman's age) is a significant determinant of the chance of pregnancy. Fig. 3.4 shows that after up to three years of

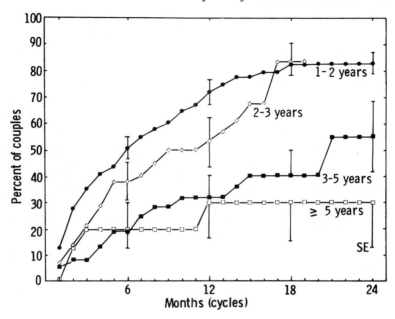

Figure 3.4 cumulative conception rates in couples with unexplained infertility, related to duration of infertility at the time they first attended the clinic. (Based on Hull *et al.* 1985.)

infertility (when first attending the clinic) the chance of conception in the next two years is not far short of normal. It seems that up to three years' failure to conceive is usually due to adversity of chance alone, and couples need only explanation and encouragement. After more than three years of unexplained infertility, and particularly after five years, the outlook is much worse (Fig. 3.4).

However, *in vitro* fertilizing capacity in couples with unexplained infertility remains normal (Wardle *et al.* 1985) and treatment by IVF offers real benefit to couples with prolonged unexplained infertility, who make up about a quarter of the whole unexplained group. If this group is added to 80 per cent of the group with tubal damage, IVF would be clearly applicable in 18 per cent of infertile couples. This would represent about 216 new couples for IVF each year per million of the general population. Of course not all couples would want IVF, but some would want to try for a second child by IVF, and research into male infertility may extend the application of IVF for both treatment and diagnosis.

I would not want to leave readers with the idea that all signposts point eventually to IVF in infertility. Ovulation induction and AID, for example, are major independent requirements, while accurate advice is all that many couples need – and such advice depends on accurate basic diagnostic methods. What is most *widely* needed is provision of good basic infertility clinics. Nevertheless, in the context of this study group it needs to be appreciated that IVF provides a powerful means of research leading to better understanding of the causes of infertility. On the other hand much research remains to be done to improve the efficiency of IVF as a treatment for infertility. Infertility is still the focus of most research with IVF.

References

Glazener, C.M.A., Kelly, N.J., Coulson, C., Lambert, P.A., Watt, E.M., Hinton, R.A., Rosevinck, B., David, J., Wier, J., Cornes, J.S., and Hull, M.G.R. (1985) The prognostic value of seminal analysis in infertility. *British Journal of Obstetrics and Gynaecology* 92: 183–84

Hull, M.G.R., Glazener, C.M.A., Kelly, N.J., Conway, D.I., Foster, P.A., Hinton, R.A., Coulson, C., Lambert, P.A., Watt, E.M., and Desai, K.M. (1985) Population study of causes, treatment, and outcome of infertility. *British Medical Journal* 291: 1693–697

Schats, R., Aitken, R.J., Templeton, A.A., and Djahanbakhch, O. (1984) The role of mucus–sperm interaction in infertility of unknown aetiology. *British Journal of Obstetrics and Gynaecology* 91: 371–76

Tietze, C. (1956) Statistical contributions to the study of human fertility. *Fertility and Sterility* 7: 88–95

Tietze, C. (1968) Fertility after discontinuation of intrauterine and oral contraception. *International Journal of Fertility* 13: 385–89

Wardle, P.G., Mitchell, J.D., McLaughlin, E.A., Ray, B.D., McDermott, A., and Hull, M.G.R. (1985) Endometriosis and ovulatory disorder: reduced fertilisation *in vitro* compared with tubal and unexplained infertility. *Lancet* 2: 236–39

Warnock, M. (Chairman) (1984) *Report of the Committee of Inquiry into Human Fertilisation and Embryology.* London: HMSO (Department of Health & Social Security) Cmnd. 9314

Discussion

Clothier: If the problem of infertility is to be used as an argument for justifying research on human pre-embryos, the missing dimension is the degree of suffering it causes.

Hull: The answer comes in anecdotal terms from all the individual couples, in the way they express their individual anguish and in the number who attend for treatment. They show the most extraordinary determination and courage in attending for all sorts of treatment, year after year, to achieve what is obviously a most powerful need. Unfortunately infertile couples tend to keep their fears bottled up. All of us here see their powerful need but the general public doesn't always see it.

Maddox: The number of 1200 per million a year quoted for the incidence of infertility is likely to be the tip of an iceberg in two senses. A lot of people may not declare themselves but in addition a lot of people may get divorced or find other partners if they don't have children. Could this question be looked at?

Hull: We should bear that in mind. It is impossible to unravel from my data.

Edwards: A study in 1969 showed that infertile couples tend to stay together rather than get divorced (Humphrey 1969). Infertility appeared to tie them together more closely, but that was sixteen years ago.

Harper: It is particularly important to measure the problems caused by infertility in an unselected population of the kind you have studied. We see a rather similar situation with couples requesting genetic counselling, who may not be typical of families with a genetic disorder in an unselected population. The kind of information one gets from people seeking referral because of infertility might by very different from that obtained from those families whom you are seeing in an unselected population. Your study appears to be ideal for measuring that kind of distress in a much more objective way than one can get from anecdotal reports.

Modell: We have a health service, not an accident service The suffering caused by infertility is a proper matter for a health service if we accept the World Health Organisation's definition of health as a state of complete mental and physical wellbeing. For most people, having children is almost the main objective of being physically and mentally well. Probably the best way to measure the suffering caused by infertility would be to ask people to assess how much satisfaction they get from having children, rather than the other way round.

Baird: When we try to assess the possible application of IVF for the treatment of infertility we obviously still lack some information. Is it known what place IVF has in the treatment of unexplained infertility of five years' duration? You showed that fertilization rates are the same in the group with unexplained fertility but did they have the same rate of pregnancies as the group with tubal disease?

Hull: One of the difficulties is to know what is meant by unexplained infertility in publications from different sources. I can only give you my definition. We don't have enough pregnancies to draw a significant conclusion yet but our pregnancy rates with IVF in unexplained infertility so far appear to match the pregnancy rates in tubal disease. Interestingly, that is not true of the pregnancy rates in male infertility or in endometriosis. I am referring to pregnancy rates per embryo. Fertilization is not the real endpoint; but successful pregnancy is more important. From the successful pregnancy rates (per embryo) it seems that there is a defect of the gamete in the egg or sperm in male infertility and in endometriosis, which further undermines the ultimate chance of success. In unexplained infertility the chance of both fertilization and pregnancy is good, but there is variable experience around the world.

Edwards: Your information is for Bristol, which is a very special area with a high standard of living. We must be wary of accepting that these estimates of infertility apply widely. A comprehensive study by the World Health Organisation recently showed that tubal disease is very prevalent in Africa (Cates, Farley, and Rowe 1985). This was due partly to infection in women and also to infection in the male. We must be careful to note the area and the community when assessing the data. These estimates refer only to one area.

Hull: I accept that, but I would guess that this information is fairly representative of this country and of similarly developed countries. It was only Africa, out of all the areas around the world that took part in the WHO study, that showed a clear difference in the tubal damage rate. The distribution of causes of infertility elsewhere was remarkably similar to those I showed.

Modell: I got the impression from your figures, Dr Hull, that perhaps up to 50 per cent of infertility might be due to genetic causes leading to sperm dysfunction.

Hull: Although genetic disorder, particularly in sperm defects and dysfunction, is significantly raised, it is identified in only a small minority of men with sperm dysfunction.

Maddox: I don't see how it is possible for infertility to be genetically inherited.

Modell: It could easily be inherited as a recessive condition.

Casey: Have you any data on the underlying causes of tubal abnormalities, since it is patients with such abnormalities who are regarded as the population suitable for IVF? I have heard the argument, which I find morally repugnant, that many of those who would be suitable for IVF are in that state because of a past induced abortion or past sexual disease. Clearly the implication when this argument is advanced is that such people should have a low priority for treatment.

Hull: That argument is about as appropriate as the punitive refusal of termination of pregnancy. Fig. 3.2 in my paper (which I didn't discuss during my talk) shows that in every group there were previous pregnancies but there were significantly more in the tubal group. Clearly pregnancy and pregnancy-related infection are an important contributor but they are not the only contributor to that particular problem. Termination of pregnancy had a significant association with coital problems. Whether the coital problems reflect a psychosexual cause or consequence of the terminated pregnancies is entirely conjectural. In the unexplained group, as you might expect, there is a significant proportion of previous children, probably because the majority of this group are essentially normal and had simply been unlucky not to have conceived (or conceived again). In every group there was a previous pregnancy but I think you are particularly interested in the data on termination. The interpretation of those data, and decisions about acceptability and appropriate treatment for related infertility, are totally different philosophical aspects.

Braude: Don't those in the group with unexplained infertility have any miscarriages?

Hull: Yes, but the figure refers to women whose *only* pregnancies had miscarried. Others who miscarried also had a pregnancy terminated or a baby, which I was primarily concerned to show. The full details are given in our paper in the *British Medical Journal* (Hull *et al.* 1985).

References

Cates, W., Farley, T.M.M., and Rowe, P.J. (1985) Worldwide patterns of infertility: is Africa different? *Lancet* 2: 596–98

Hull, M.G.R., Glazener, C.M.A., Kelly, N.J., Conway, D.I., Foster, P.A., Hinton, R.A., Coulson, C., Lambert, P.A., Watt, E.M., and Desai, K.M. (1985) Population study of causes, treatment, and outcome of infertility. *British Medical Journal* 291: 1693–697

Humphrey, M. (1969) *The Hostage Seekers: A Study of Childless and Adopting Couples.* London: Longman

FOUR

Clinical aspects of in vitro fertilization

R.G. Edwards

I have tried to present an up-to-date analysis of the clinical aspects of *in vitro* fertilization, indicating where new knowledge might help to improve the method or introduce new forms of treatment. Research is needed on many aspects of the procedure, including forms of hormonal stimulation, the culture of embryos, implantation, and luteal phase support. Children born after this procedure do not seem to have more abnormalities than children conceived *in vivo*, although more information is needed. New procedures are rapidly being introduced.

This chapter on the technological aspects of *in vitro* fertilization includes descriptions of follicular stimulation, the induction of follicular maturation, collection of oocytes, fertilization and cleavage *in vitro*, implantation, embryo mortality after implantation, deliveries, and birth (for further references see Edwards *et al.* 1984; Edwards, Purdy, and Steptoe 1985). First, however, I shall briefly describe the normal menstrual cycle in order to compare it with the stimulated cycles used for *in vitro* fertilization.

The natural menstrual cycle

Three phases of the natural menstrual cycle can be distinguished. The onset of menstruation signals the onset of the *follicular phase* of a cycle, when several follicles start to expand under the influence of follicle-stimulating hormone (FSH) (Fig. 4.1). Usually, one follicle becomes dominant after a few days and completes its growth while the others regress. Occasionally, two or more follicles can grow at the same rate, which leads to the ovulation of two or more oocytes and (if these are fertilized) to the formation of dizygotic twins, triplets, etc. The follicular phase lasts about twelve to fourteen days (Fig. 4.1). It is controlled by FSH and luteinizing hormone (LH) from the pituitary gland, FSH and LH themselves being regulated by hypothalamic LH-releasing hormone (LHRH) and feedback systems from the ovary involving oestrogen and inhibin.

On day thirteen of the cycle, or thereabouts, a surge of LH and FSH induces the *preovulatory phase*. The oocyte begins its maturation preparatory to ovulation and fertilization. The follicle enlarges rapidly and ruptures at ovulation, liberating the oocyte into the oviduct.

The ruptured follicle is rapidly filled with cells and forms the corpus luteum. This gland releases oestrogen and progesterone, which dominate the third phase of the cycle, the *luteal phase*. The combination of these steroid hormones induces changes in the oviduct which sustain the cleaving embryo; the combination also induces changes in the uterus, which becomes secretory and able to accept an implanting embryo. If implantation does not occur, the corpus luteum degenerates on day twenty-eight or thereabouts and its secretion of steroid hormones declines. Much of the progesterone-dependent endometrium (the mucous membrane lining the uterus) is then sloughed away, resulting in menstruation. If an embryo has implanted, its secretions – notably human chorionic gonadotropin (hCG) – sustain the corpus luteum, which maintains the uterus in its secretory state, prevents menstruation, and so supports the embryo through its early growth.

Follicular stimulation for *in vitro* fertilization

Virtually all patients attending for *in vitro* fertilization receive some form of stimulation in order to stimulate the growth of follicles which would otherwise degenerate. The natural menstrual cycle is rarely used, because there is a higher chance of

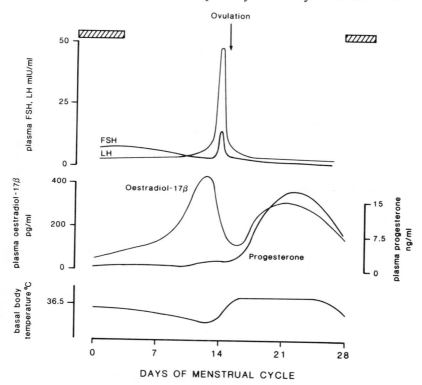

Figure 4.1 the fluctuating levels of gonadotropins (LH, FSH) and steroids (oestrogens, progesterone) during the menstrual cycle. The onset of menstruation (hatched bars) signifies the beginning of the menstrual cycle. Rising levels of oestrogens in the follicular (first) phase of the cycle trigger the surge of LH and FSH, which introduce the preovulatory phase and ovulation. The formation of the corpus luteum results in the secretion of oestrogen (oestradiol-17β) and progesterone typical of the luteal phase, which ends when menstruation starts again

implantation if two or more embryos can be replaced than if only one is replaced. Until recently, either clomiphene (a weak oestrogen) or human menopausal gondadotropins (HMG, a mixture of FSH and LH) were used as follicle stimulants, but a combination of clomiphene and HMG now appears to be better than either of these substances alone, as the combination leads to the recovery of three or more preovulatory oocytes in many patients. Clomiphene has both oestrogenic and anti-oestrogenic effects and stimulates the release of FSH and LH from the pituitary gland. Other new methods have also been introduced, e.g. the use of pure FSH instead of HMG (Jones *et al.* 1982), and LHRH agonists (Fleming *et al.* 1982), which inactivates the patient's own pituitary gland, followed by HMG.

The combination of clomiphene and HMG may be given from day two or later in the menstrual cycle. The timing of HMG is also variable and we currently begin giving daily injections (100 international units) from day five.

Follicle growth is assessed by measuring oestrogen levels in the plasma or urine and by examining follicles ultrasonically (Kratochwil, Urban, and Friedrich 1972). Follicles are scanned every second or third day and this is the only method of follicular assessment used in some clinics. We rely equally on endocrine data. Frequent ultrasonic scanning of the ovary appears to be harmless, but care is needed in interpreting these observations because follicular size is not necessarily a true indication of follicular maturity.

The combination of clomiphene and HMG is a powerful stimulant, resulting in the development of several follicles and high levels of oestrogens in most patients. These high levels are compatible with pregnancy, but the hyperstimulation of many follicles can lead to disorders in follicular growth and to premature luteinization and abnormal fertilization.

The induction of follicular and oocyte maturation

Some patients given follicular stimulants discharge their own surge of LH and FSH in mid-cycle, which stimulates the maturation of follicles and oocytes. Most patients do not have an LH surge, despite having several large follicles and high levels of oestrogens; perhaps the secretion of inhibin and other inhibitors from these follicles interferes with secretion from the pituitary gland (Hodgen 1982). These patients are given hCG to induce maturation before their follicles degenerate. All patients must be monitored closely since a major problem lies in identifying those who have their own LH surge.

Repeated assays of LH in all patients are therefore needed each day and simplified methods of assay are essential. The fluorescent linked immunoassay (Delfia, LKB) that we now use is rapid and can be read within two hours; one person can set up 100 assays each day.

Major difficulties can arise in patients who have weak LH surges after they have been given follicle stimulants. Indeed, some LH surges are so weak that they may be overlooked, and hCG may be mistakenly administered after the preovulatory changes have begun. This can result in luteinized follicles being found at laparoscopy and to abnormal fertilization (Edwards 1985a). Rising levels of progesterone in the follicular phase also indicate that ovulation is approaching. Nearly 90 per cent of patients reach this stage of their treatment. The reasons for discharging the others include weak follicle growth, unbalanced hormones, premature ejaculation, and failure to identify a weak LH surge.

Collection of oocytes

Laparoscopy, which allows many preovulatory oocytes to be recovered from their follicles (Steptoe and Edwards 1970; Steptoe and Webster 1982), undoubtedly paved the way for the introduction of *in vitro* fertilization. Ultrasound, which can be used without general anaesthesia, has been introduced recently for follicular aspiration (Lenz and Lauritsen 1982; Wikland *et al.* 1983) and the success rates approach those obtained with laparoscopy. In this method follicle contents are aspirated and the follicle is flushed out until the oocyte is recovered.

There is debate about whether a damaged oviduct should be closed off during oocyte collection or during a preliminary laparoscopy. Embryos placed in the uterus might enter such enlarged oviducts and develop into ectopic pregnancies. This condition has occurred in many clinics and is perhaps the most serious clinical problem associated with *in vitro* fertilization.

Very high rates of oocyte recovery are now achieved in most clinics, and 95 per cent or more patients can expect one or more preovulatory oocytes to be aspirated. This part of the treatment is perhaps the most successful of all aspects of *in vitro* fertilization.

Fertilization *in vitro*

Oocytes are normally aspirated between two and four hours before ovulation is expected, and a similar delay is needed before they are inseminated. Part of this time is required for sperm capacitation (see below), and inseminations are usually performed between one and six hours after oocyte collection (Edwards, Steptoe, and Purdy 1980; Trounson *et al.* 1982). Some clinics use a standard interval between oocyte collection and insemination; others, including ourselves, rely on the state of viscosity of the cumulus cells around the oocytes. An interval of many hours is not incompatible with fertilization and development of a foetus to full term. Various attempts have been made to assess oocyte maturity with non-invasive methods, without much success. Information about maturation is sadly lacking in human oocytes, although oocytes that are relatively immature when collected can complete their maturation *in vitro* and develop into full-term babies (Veeck *et al.* 1983).

Several media are used for fertilization and embryonic growth *in vitro* (Edwards 1985b). We use sperm suspensions containing 2–20×10^5/ml, depending on the 'quality' of the sperm sample, to inseminate oocytes in droplets of medium held beneath liquid paraffin, under a gas phase of 5 per cent carbon dioxide in air. Other clinics use small tubes or open dishes for culturing oocytes and embryos.

Sperm penetration into the oocytes begins two to three hours after insemination. The interval presumably represents the period needed for capacitation to occur, although very little is known about the capacitation of human spermatozoa (Ahuja 1985). More than 85 per cent of preovulatory oocytes from patients with tubal disorders are fertilized *in vitro*, provided that the spermatozoa are 'satisfactory' (Cohen *et al.* 1984) (Table 4.1). This group of patients can serve as a control for others, because most of the men do not have fertility problems.

After fertilization, most eggs contain two pronuclei, but the use of follicular stimulants increases the incidence of eggs with three

Table 4.1   Fertilization rates at Bourn
Hall in 1984, for various forms of
infertility

indication	proportion of patients with one or more fertilized eggs (%)	
tubal	634/659	(95.2)
idiopathic	46/54	(85.2)
male infertility	36/60	(58.3)
immunological	18/20	(90.0)
endometriosis	12/14	(85.7)
cervical	21/23	(91.3)
other	41/44	(93.2)

pronuclei to about 5 per cent. These eggs have presumably been fertilized by two spermatozoa, that is they are dispermic. Dispermic eggs are also found if luteinization occurs before laparoscopy; ovarian hyperstimulation might cause the oocytes in dominant follicles to become overripe because maturation is inhibited if the LH surge is suppressed (Hodgen 1982). Dispermy might also arise through the premature stimulation of secondary follicles, as their oocytes may fail to develop a full defence against polyspermy (Soupart and Strong 1975; Mohr and Trounson 1982).

High rates of fertilization are possible with oocytes and spermatozoa from patients with various disorders. Many couples have more than one cause of infertility between them (Tables 4.1 and 4.2). Conditions such as viscous seminal plasma or small amounts of cells and debris in semen do not depress the chances of fertilization. Reduced motility, massive clumping or tail agglutination of spermatozoa, and, worst of all, large amounts of cells or debris in semen, presumably due to inflammation, can impair fertilization. Nevertheless, lack of spermatozoa (oligospermia) and idiopathic infertility can be successfully treated by *in vitro* fertilization (Cohen *et al.* 1984) (Tables 4.1 and 4.2), and many pregnancies have been established by this method when male infertility had previously been intractable.

More research is needed on methods of sperm preparation in cases of male infertility. Low rates of fertilization can be achieved

Table 4.2   Male and mixed infertility (Cohen *et al.* 1984 and unpublished)

	male factor only	female and male factors
no. of couples	60	89
age	33	34
infertility (years)	6.5	7.8
fertilizations per cycle	66%	80%
pregnancies per laparascopy	22%	17%
pregnancies per replacement	33%	22%
infertility of pregnant patients (years)	6.7	8.7

provided sufficient oocytes are available, despite the presence of seemingly major obstacles in unsatisfactory sperm samples. The very simple methods of layering and 'swim-up' have given astonishingly good results, and other methods in which a spermatozoon is microinjected beneath the zona pellucida of the ovum might give further improvements.

The introduction of a procedure called GIFT (gamete intra-Fallopian tube transfer), in which spermatozoa are placed in the oviduct of suitable patients instead of being fertilized *in vitro*, will simplify the procedure for some patients. About 25 per cent of patients deliver one or more children when four oocytes are replaced (Asch 1985).

Cleavage *in vitro*

Different types of media supplemented with various levels of human serum and albumin have been used to support cleaving embryos. The human embryo can evidently tolerate a wide variety of media but not enough is known about the metabolic needs of the embryo for better media to be prepared. A better understanding of the requirements of the human embryo could be a major benefit for *in vitro* fertilization. We already know, for example, that more pyruvate is taken up by human embryos than by mouse embryos (Leese *et al.* 1986).

The growth of human embryos capable of developing to

blastocysts, as assessed from their morphology or the number of nuclei, does not appear to be seriously impaired *in vitro* compared with development *in vivo*. Nevertheless in some embryos growth *in vitro* is arrested during cleavage, and this may occur at various stages of development from the two-cell stage to the morula (early blastocyst) (Fishel *et al.* 1985). We do not know whether these embryos are metabolically abnormal or whether the failure is a consequence of follicular stimulation or of the conditions of culture *in vitro*; nor do we know whether an abnormal chromosome complement is responsible: embryos with three pronuclei, which are presumably the precursors of triploid embryos, develop just as well as those with two pronuclei. Some embryos may cleave rapidly under certain circumstances, e.g. after delayed fertilization, whereas others fail to cleave at all or become degenerate.

Several clinics are now trying to type preimplantation embryos for inherited defects. This will be achieved by taking one or two morula cells (blastomeres) for typing two-cell, four-cell or eight-cell embryos, or by excising a small piece of trophoblast (Edwards 1985a). Several DNA probes for various inherited conditions are now available, but the methods of hybridization *in situ* will have to be improved to suit the small amount of tissue available.

Implantation

A critical feature of *in vitro* fertilization is the incidence of implantation after the replacement of one or more embryos. We replace a maximum of three embryos except in patients with numerous failures, when four are replaced. Some clinics replace more, even up to sixteen at a single replacement.

Results from Bourn Hall since the opening of the clinic are shown in Table 4.3, which gives clinical pregnancies only, all short-lived pregnancies characterized by transitory rises in hCG (biochemical pregnancies) being excluded. Every patient admitted since Bourn Hall opened is included in this table. Many of them have defects such as short luteal phases, endometriosis, fibroids, etc. Some patients included in this table have returned repeatedly without success; hence these figures include patients with major difficulties in even achieving implantation. The

Table 4.3   Incidence of implantation (%)[a]

embryos replaced	patients aged	
	under 40 (n = 2644)	40 + (n = 267)
1	15.0	10.7
2	23.0	10.8
3	30.7	19.3
All	24.3	14.2

[a]Only clinical pregnancies are included, all biochemical pregnancies being omitted (see text).

Table 4.4   Implantation in patients of all ages, with various forms of infertility, at Bourn Hall in 1984

indication	no. of embryos replaced		
	1	2	3
tubal	12/80	23/108	139/438
idiopathic	1/5	3/13	10/28
male infertility	1/8	2/11	4/16
immunological	0/3	1/4	4/11
endometriosis	1/4	1/10	10/23
cervical	2/4	3/5	5/12
other	0/3	0/11	8/26

Data show the proportion of patients with clinical pregnancies.

incidence of implantation is high compared with the incidence at other clinics, surpassing 30 per cent after the replacement of three embryos in patients under forty years of age. This rate has been maintained for three or four years. Implantation rates are similar in patients with different forms of infertility (Table 4.4). Once fertilization has occurred, the chances of pregnancy therefore seem to be similar whatever the original cause of infertility.

Many attempts have been made to increase the chances of implantation. The use of different culture media, or modifications in the technique of replacement, have not led to any significant improvement since the initial work in Oldham. Improvements are obviously necessary, since fewer than 20 per cent of the replaced embryos implant. This rate of implantation is lower than after conception *in vivo*, when about 25 per cent of embryos implant. The reduced chance of implantation after embryo replacement might not be due solely to embryonic factors; uterine factors or abnormal endocrine systems in women given follicular stimulants may also be responsible. Many clinics have tried to raise the chances of implantation by using progesterone or hCG to support the luteal phase. Such support might be helpful since the secretion of hCG-β from trophoblast outgrowths is lower than that of trophoblastic cells of embryos conceived *in vivo* (Fishel, Edwards, and Evans 1984). Our own attempts have not had much success. HCG will rescue a corpus luteum which is almost extinct and is secreting very low levels of progesterone. Nevertheless, controlled trials have failed to reveal any benefit, even in our best series of patients, and we are now testing other forms of luteal support.

Are there any clinical clues to the low rate of implantation? Abnormal forms of implantation after embryo replacement include delayed implantation (assessed by a delayed rise in levels of hCG), ectopic implantation, blighted ova, molar pregnancies (tumorous growths), and biochemical pregnancies (Edwards 1985b). A delay in implantation implies that the implantation 'window' is open for several days, and considerable progress could be made if methods were found to widen this window after *in vitro* fertilization. The incidence of ectopic pregnancies appears to be related to the number of embryos replaced.

Several clinics have begun to freeze embryos for storage (Mohr and Trounson 1983; Zeilmaker *et al.* 1984; Cohen *et al.* 1985). We have been testing the respective advantages of freezing cleaving embryos, using dimethyl sulphoxide, or of freezing blastocysts, using glycerol (Ashwood-Smith 1986). Blastocysts survive better but there are fewer available for freezing, since many cleaving embryos do not reach this stage of development. Improved methods of freezing oocytes and embryos could offer great advantages, and this is now a very active area of research.

Embryo mortality after implantation

Many women abort after *in vitro* fertilization, the incidence appearing to be higher than after conception *in vivo*. Unfortunately, there are no strict comparisons yet between IVF patients whose average age is thirty-five and patients conceiving *in vivo*. Some authorities suggest that many embryos also die after conception *in vivo* (Edmonds *et al*. 1982) but the incidence of abortion appears to be greater with *in vitro* fertilization, implying that more foetuses are abnormal or that implantation was impaired. Some studies of embryos conceived *in vitro* have indicated that many such embryos have chromosomal anomalies (e.g. Angell *et al*. 1983), but it is possible that highly anomalous forms such as haploids might arise as a consequence of treatments practised in particular clinics. Anomalies in the site of implantation do not appear to be the cause of abortions. Scans of singleton, twin and triplet foetuses conceived *in vitro* have shown that all were implanted in the fundal region (G. Anderson, personal communications).

The high incidence of abortion after *in vitro* fertilization is associated partly with the previous obstetric history of the patient (Table 4.5); patients with an abnormal history have a much higher chance of abortion. This indicates that maternal factors are important in causing abortion. Patients with no previous obstetric history have the same or a better chance of implantation and a lower rate of abortion than those with a previous pregnancy (Table 4.5).

Many foetuses 'vanish' during pregnancy, with a triplet gestation becoming a singleton or a twin, or a twin pregnancy becoming a singleton. About 18 per cent of foetuses vanish in *in vitro*-fertilized pregnancies known to be twin or triplet during gestation (Edwards 1985b). Not enough is known about foetuses conceived *in vivo* to say whether this value is higher or lower than after natural conception.

Deliveries and births

The evidence of deliveries and births after *in vitro* fertilization is reassuring so far, for there is no increase in difficulties at

Table 4.5 Implantation and abortion in relation to previous obstetric history

previous history	implantation						abortion
	one[a]		*two[a]*		*three[a]*		*all pregnancies combined, % aborting*
	no.	% pregnant	no.	% pregnant	no.	% pregnant	
none	85	20.0	40	35.0	23	34.8	17.9
full-term delivery	91	17.6	51	29.4	55	38.1	17.3
complications	307	19.2	158	20.9	167	30.0	33.1

[a] No. of embryos replaced.

Table 4.6 Deliveries after embryo replacement at Bourn Hall in patients younger than 40

embryos	% of patients delivering after different treatments				
	clom/ LH	clom/ HCG	clom/ HMG/LH	clom/ HMG/HCG	all
1	10.0	8.5	5.5	15.9	10.1
2	19.0	17.9	17.2	13.4	16.6
3	19.5	13.0	19.1	24.2	22.7
all	13.8	13.7	15.0	21.5	17.7

Total number of deliveries = 469.
clom = clomiphene.

parturition, or in the incidence of abnormal babies compared with the incidence after conception *in vivo*. After various forms of follicular stimulation almost a quarter of the patients under forty years of age deliver one or more children when three embryos are replaced (see Table 4.6); this is most encouraging since it is greater than the incidence of births after natural conception (Steptoe, Edwards, and Walters 1986). With patients over forty years of age, the number of deliveries is greatly reduced. For many couples receiving one or two embryos the problem is male infertility, and the number of embryos replaced is less because their chance of fertilization is reduced.

Table 4.7 Incidence of multiple births (figures from Bourn Hall)

	embryos replaced	
	2	3
no. of births	109	285
no. of twins	18	59
no. of triplets	0	12
no. of babies	127	368
% increase[a]	16.5	26.3

[a] No. of twins or twins and triplets/no. of births.

The incidence of multiple births in patients receiving two or three embryos in Bourn Hall is shown in Table 4.7. Many twins and triplets have implanted or been born, not all of them included in this table. The incidence of multiple pregnancy and births is much lower in other clinics, despite the replacement of more than three embryos. This variation between clinics could be due to the use of different methods of embryo culture. The overall incidence of children born in Bourn Hall is therefore much higher than the number of deliveries; when three embryos are replaced, about thirty children are born for each 100 replacements (Steptoe *et al.* 1986).

Many patients who conceived by *in vitro* fertilization in our clinic are delivered by Caesarian section, presumably due to concern by gynaecologists for these high-risk infertile patients. A few children have been born prematurely, especially those in triplet pregnancies. Four major abnormalities have occurred among more than 500 children conceived *in vitro*, some of these perhaps being inherited (Table 4.8). Two of the four were treated successfully at birth. Many of the minor abnormalities also appear to be inherited. So far, only about half of the babies have been fully assessed by the Medical Research Council, with whom we are collaborating. The incidence of anomalies does not appear to be greater than after conception *in vivo* but it is too early to draw any conclusions on the exact incidence of abnormal babies conceived *in vitro*.

Table 4.8   Anomalies among 500 births after treatment at Bourn Hall

major anomalies (1 each)	minor anomalies (1 each unless indicated)
minor hydrocephalus of twin[a] Russel Silber dwarf (one of twins) tracheal sling[a] cleft right hand	talipes (2) syndactyly of toes vitiligo temporary systolic murmur persistent systolic murmur hypospadies elevated nasal septum

[a] treated surgically.

Acknowledgements

I am deeply indebted to many colleagues at Bourn Hall, especially Patrick Steptoe, for permission to quote from previous publications based on work there.

References

Ahuja, K. (1985) In I.W.H. Johnston (ed.) *Proceedings of the Fourth World Congress on In Vitro Fertilization and Embryo Transfer, Melbourne, 1985.* New York: Plenum Press, in press.

Angell, R.R., Aitken, R.J., Van Look, P.F.A., Lumsden, M.A., and Templeton, A.A. (1983) Chromosome abnormalities in human embryos after *in vitro* fertilization. *Nature* 303: 336–38

Asch, R. (1985) In I.W.H. Johnston (ed.) *Proceedings of the Fourth World Congress on In Vitro Fertilization and Embryo Transfer, Melbourne, 1985.* New York: Plenum Press, in press.

Ashwood-Smith, M.J. (1986) Cryopreservation procedures do not present genetic hazards. *Human Reproduction* 1: supplement 1, A34.

Cohen, J., Edwards, R.G., Fehilly, C.B., Fishel, S.B., Hewitt, J., Purdy, J., Rowland, G.F., Steptoe, P.C., and Webster, J. (1984) *In vitro* fertilization: a treatment for male infertility. *Fertility and Sterility* 43: 422–32

Cohen, J., Simons, R.F., Edwards, R.G., Fehilly, B., and Fishel, S.B. (1985) Pregnancies following the frozen storage of expanding human blastocysts. *Journal of In Vitro Fertilization and Embryo Transfer* 2: 59–64

Edmonds, D.K., Lindsay, K.S., Miller, J.F., Williamson, E., and Wood, P.J. (1982) Early embryonic mortality in women. *Fertility and Sterility* 38: 447–53

Edwards, R.G. (1985a) Current status of human conception *in vitro*. *Proceedings of the Royal Society of London B Biological Sciences* 223: 417–48

Edwards, R.G. (1985b) Normal and abnormal implantation in the human uterus. In R.G. Edwards, J.M. Purdy and P.C. Steptoe (eds) *Implantation of the Human Embryo*. London: Academic Press

Edwards, R.G., Steptoe, P.C., and Purdy, J.M. (1980) Establishing full-term human pregnancies using cleaving embryos grown *in vitro*. *British Journal of Obstetrics and Gynaecology* 87: 737–56

Edwards, R.G., Fishel, S.B., Cohen, J., Fehilly, C.B., Purdy, J.M., Slater, J.H., Steptoe, P.C., and Webster, J.M. (1984) Factors influencing the success of *in vitro* fertilization for alleviating human infertility. *Journal of In Vitro Fertilization and Embryo Transfer* 1: 3–23

Edwards, R.G., Purdy, J.M., and Steptoe, P.C. (1985) *Implantation of the Human Embryo*. London: Academic Press

Fishel, S.B., Edwards, R.G., and Evans, C.J. (1984) Human chorionic gonadotrophin secreted by preimplantation embryos cultured *in vitro*. *Science* 223: 816–18

Fishel, S.B., Cohen, J., Fehilly, C.B., Purdy, J.M., and Edwards, R.G. (1985) Factors influencing human embryonic development *in vitro*. In M. Seppälä and R.G. Edwards (eds) *In Vitro* Fertilization and Embryo Transfer. *Annals of the New York Academy of Sciences*, vol. 442: part VII

Fleming, R., Adam, A.H., Barlow, D.H., Black, W.P., MacNaughton, M.C., and Coutts, J.R. (1982) A new systematic treatment for infertile women with abnormal hormone profiles. *British Journal of Obstetrics and Gynaecology* 89: 80–83

Hodgen, G.D. (1982) The dominant ovarian follicle. *Fertility and Sterility* 38: 281–300

Jones, H.W., Jones, G.S., Andres, M.C., Acosta, A., Bundren, C., Garcia, J., Sandow, B., Veeck, L., Wilkes, C., Witmyer, J., Wortham, E., and Wright, G. (1982) The program for *in vitro* fertilization at Norfolk. *Fertility and Sterility* 38: 14–21

Kratochwil, A., Urban, G., and Friedrich, F. (1972) Ultrasonic tomography of the ovaries. *Annales Chirurgiae et Gynecologiae Fenniae* 61: 211–14

Leese, H.J., Hooper, M.A.K., Edwards, R.G., and Ashwood-Smith, M.J. (1986) Uptake of pyruvate by early human embryos determined by a non-invasive technique. *Human Reproduction* 3: 181–82

Lenz, S., and Lauritsen, J.G. (1982) Ultrasonically guided percutaneous aspiration of human follicles under local anaesthesia. *Fertility and Sterility* 38: 673–77

Mohr, L. and Trounson, A.O. (1982) Comparative ultrastructure of hatched human, mouse and bovine blastocysts. *Journal of Reproduction and Fertility* 66: 499–504

Mohr, L. and Trounson, A.O. (1983) Human pregnancy following cryopreservation, thawing and transfer of an eight-cell embryo. *Nature* 305: 707–709

Soupart, P. and Strong, P.A. (1975) Ultrastructural observations on polyspermic penetrations of zona pellucida-free human oocytes inseminated *in vitro. Fertility and Sterility* 26: 523–37

Steptoe, P.C. and Edwards, R.G. (1970) Laparoscopic recovery of preovulatory human oocytes after priming of ovaries with gonadotrophins. *Lancet* 1: 683–89

Steptoe, P.C. and Webster, J. (1982) Laparoscopy of the normal and disordered ovary. In R.G. Edwards and J.M. Purdy (eds) *Human Conception In Vitro*. London: Academic Press, pp. 97–103

Steptoe, P.C., Edwards, R.G., and Walters, D.E. (1986) Observations on 767 clinical pregnancies and 500 births after human *in vitro* fertilization. *Human Reproduction* 2: 89–94

Trounson, A.O., Mohr, L.R., Wood, C., and Leeton, J.F. (1982) Effect of delayed insemination on *in vitro* fertilization, culture and transfer of human embryos. *Journal of Reproduction and Fertility* 64: 285–94

Veeck, L.L., Wortham, J.W., Jr., Witmyer, J., Sandow, B.A., Acosta, A.A., Garcia, J.E., Jones, G.S., and Jones, H.W., Jr. (1983) Maturation and fertilization of morphologically immature human oocytes in a program of *in vitro* fertilization. *Fertility and Sterility* 39: 594–602

Wikland, M., Nilsson, L., Hansson, R., Hamberger, L., and Janson, P.O. (1983) Collection of human oocytes by the use of sonography. *Fertility and Sterility* 39: 603–08

Zeilmaker, G.H., Alberda, A.T., van Gent, I., Rykmans, C.M.P.M., Diendigh, A.C. (1984) Two pregnancies following transfer of intact frozen–thawed embryos. *Fertility and Sterility* 42: 293–96

Discussion

Clothier: Which areas of research on pre-embryos would you particularly like to see go forward, and why, Dr Edwards?

Edwards: Mostly those connected with the treatment itself. For example, we know very little about the metabolism of the human embryo. We have done some studies but we need to know much more. We need detailed chromosomal analysis of embryos conceived *in vitro*, because we have no idea of the true incidence of anomalies. We do not have such data *in vivo* either and we have to make estimates from abortion rates. It could be a great advance if we could get 100 per cent of our embryos to blastocysts. I would feel then that we were getting it right.

Lock: You have obviously had to make some very difficult and controversial decisions. Can you tell us something about your ethics committee?

Edwards: When we started in the 1960s there were very few ethical committees in the UK of the sort we know today. We asked the Oldham General Hospital to assess our work in their committee in the early 1970s, and we followed their guidelines from then until 1978. When Bourn Hall opened in 1980, we attempted to establish an ethical committee within eighteen months, with people from the Cambridge area. At present we have a scientist, a professor of law, a bishop, a former mistress of a Cambridge women's college, a gynaecologist, a chairman who is a general practitioner, and a secretary who holds science and theology degrees. We ask them to advise on virtually everything we do, and only a few minor decisions are taken in the laboratory.

Rodeck: We heard earlier that some 70 per cent of spontaneous conceptions are lost and you were a bit sceptical about that. Doesn't it seem that the failure rate with IVF is very similar?

Edwards: The losses after IVF are very similar to the estimates for losses after conception *in vivo*. I have to question the estimates for embryonic death *in vivo* made by Edmonds (Edmonds *et al.* 1982) and by others. They are based on transient rises in levels of human chorionic gonadotropin (hCG). Such transient rises are rare in our work in Bourn Hall, occurring in a maximum of some 15 per cent of all conceptions. The rises reported by others may be due to some cause other than pregnancy. We need to know more about the population under study, how often intercourse takes place, and so on. Nevertheless, some embryos are lost very early after natural conception, so the ethical point about such early mortality must be accepted. We need more data on the real losses and the time of occurrence.

Braude: What else can those rises in hCG mean, other than trophoblast activity?

Edwards: We must ensure first that the assay techniques are highly specific and secondly that there is no other reason for the rise in hCG. For example, was hCG assessed throughout the luteal phase? Are there any other conditions after a failure of implantation when hCG might be produced in some other tissue?

Jacobs: I can shed some light on abortion rates, based on a very controlled system where we induce ovulation in women with amenorrhoea. As Mike Hull pointed out, there is a very good prognosis when luteinizing hormone releasing hormone (LHRH) is used with very careful ultrasound monitoring right through the cycle. We can date ovulation and follow events right through the luteal phase into early pregnancy. In patients with simple hypothalamic pituitary lesions who are monitored in this way the abortion rate is 10–12 per cent. In women with polycystic ovary disease the abortion rate is 50 per cent, using exactly the same criteria. There is therefore no single answer to the question about the rate of spontaneous abortions.

Baird: There has been a lot of cricitism of Keith Edmonds' paper (Edmonds *et al.* 1982). This study was of healthy women trying to get pregnant in the Southampton area, compared with sterilized women who had a similar frequency of intercourse. The basal level of hCG that Edmonds and co-workers used was the maximum amount they detected in the control (sterilized) women. The methods used for the study satisfied the referees of a major scientific journal.

There is preliminary evidence that a significant proportion of embryos fertilized *in vitro* have lethal chromosome abnormalities (Angell *et al.* 1983). This work, which was done in Edinburgh by Ros Evans, has recently been updated. The proportion of abnormal embryos is about 30 per cent. This study shows that a significant minority of embryos fertilized *in vitro* do not have the capacity to develop further even if they are replaced. These embryos are indistinguishable morphologically, on conventional criteria, from those that go on to form a pregnancy. In treatment programmes, therefore, some 30 per cent of embryos will not survive.

Edwards: I have always had reservations about data from IVF because there is a great deal of variation between success rates in different clinics. The quality of the embryology may make a great difference. We must be careful about drawing conclusions from one clinic and one set of conditions. We need results from a wide variety of clinics.

Rodeck: This is very important when we assess success rates. We need to know how many losses in IVF pregnancies are due to abnormalities which could not be reduced by improvements in techniques for IVF. At the moment there are no means of deciding what proportion of the embryos lost before implantation are abnormal chromosomally. However, if chromosome analysis were done on the aborted material a lot of information could be gained from women who have had IVF and who abort clinically detected pregnancies. These women are highly motivated to find out whether what they have lost is abnormal. It is difficult to get this information from the general population because women often abort at home and the conceptus is lost or becomes contaminated so that it cannot be cultured.

McLaren: It is very important to be able to assess the normality of the cleavage stage that is put back into the woman. One needs to know not only whether there are any chromosomal defects but also whether there is any other abnormality. Two-cell and eight-cell stages in mice sometimes look obviously abnormal but often they look perfectly normal. We cannot tell which are good and which are bad, yet we know that some have no future after implantation. Bob, you showed us that cleavage stopped at different stages – two cells, four cells, and so on. Have you done any prospective studies on cleavage stages, in the sense of predicting which will stop developing and which will survive? The morphological appearance is an extremely crude measure. It must be very difficult when you are dealing with human patients to have to decide which three morulae out of six you are going to put back. We need research to devise a more objective method of assessment.

Edwards: I fully agree. We keep detailed records of cleavage in the embryos and the numbers replaced. We obviously select the best three we can. Fortunately the number of times we find three embryos all with fragments is not high, and we have had pregnancies with the most unusual-looking embryos.

Dunstan: If chromosomally defective embryos are morphologically indistinguishable from normal embryos what methods will show which kind is which without destroying the embryo? And will those methods leave the embryo viable for reimplantation if you find it in order?

Edwards: Eggs with three pronuclei are almost certainly dispermic, although some may arise because a polar body is incorporated into the egg. They are almost certainly the precursors of triploid embryos, hydatidiform moles or other forms of anomalous growth. About 3 to 5 per cent of fertilized eggs are like this, and we exclude them from freezing or replacement. Of course to exclude those we have first to examine the pronuclear content of all fertilized eggs. We can see the pronuclei under a low-power microscope so there is no difficulty in recognizing them.

Dunstan: This examination does not damage the embryo?

Edwards: No, not usually. We do our best not to damage the embryo. We might have to dissect the remaining cumulus cells from around the egg with fine needles and occasionally some eggs are damaged in this procedure.

For continued growth, we really need to know whether an embryo is genetically normal, which is almost impossible to find out. More immediately, we may be able to find out whether embryos are metabolizing normally.

Leese and his colleagues have measured the uptake of pyruvate, glucose, and lactate in cleaving mouse embryos (Leese and Barton 1984). The results agree with results found using radioactive tracers.

We have repeated the work in the human embryo and can measure the uptake of pyruvate without any difficulty (Leese *et al*. 1986). Moreover, this can be done without damage in embryos which are later replaced in the mother or frozen for later replacement, so large-scale studies are possible. We have to analyse the medium from around the egg, after a specific time. The shift to glucose incorporation would probably be a very significant step in metabolism. Whether these techniques can ever be used to identify the abnormal embryos or the best embryos for replacement remains to be seen. These are all non-invasive procedures.

Baird: In general terms, to evaluate the predictive value of such a test it would be enormously advantageous to be able to study the embryo experimentally rather than to have to replace it. If you could predict, by measuring some constituent released into the culture medium, which embryos had forty-seven chromosomes, you would not know whether that was really so until you looked at the embryo's chromosomes – but if you put the embryo back in the mother you would never be able to find that out.

Williamson: At present no non-invasive technique for looking for DNA defects before eight weeks or so has been tested. We shall be discussing this later on.

Harper: Is the low level of abnormalities in your series likely to be due to the women taking special care, Professor Edwards, or are they from high socioeconomic groups that might be at lower risk? Or do you perhaps screen out people who might have family histories of particular problems?

Edwards: Our assessment is not yet complete so we cannot be sure about the exact incidence of anomalies at birth. Our patients are probably from the higher socioeconomic groups but they are also older than the average (a mean of thirty-five years). I doubt that there is any selective abortion due to our choosing particular kinds of embryos for replacement. We choose three out of four or five, but sometimes from as many as ten embryos. The only exclusions are those eggs with three pronuclei, and perhaps those cleaving slightly more slowly. We exclude the tripronucleate eggs and freeze the slow-growing embryos.

Harper: In genetic counselling when we quote a normal population or background figure for genetic risk it is usually 2 per cent for something serious and 3–4 per cent including the trivial defects. Maybe for couples who have no adverse factors we should be quoting rather lower figures.

Iglesias: It is true, as was stated earlier, that many women and couples suffer because of their infertility. I find it puzzling that very little is done to *prevent* infertility. Preventive medicine is a concern of the medical profession; why not so in this field?

I should like to ask Professor Edwards a question. From contacts with people working on IVF in other European countries I have heard the theory that it is possible to have a clinically safe programme of *in vitro* fertilization without having to destroy some human embryos deliberately. I am not sure of this. For without experiments on a certain number of embryos, how could the best culture medium and the other conditions for generating embryos be determined? The question arises even in the most stringent case of the married couples seeking *in vitro* fertilization with their own gametes, and where practitioners are prepared to transfer all the embryos they generate. So, is it possible to have a good clinical programme without destroying some embryos (including the abnormal ones which are now not transferred), so that some other embryos may survive and a child may be born?

Edwards: I avoid using the word 'experiment'. A clinic would probably be quite happy if it could sustain the cleavage of embryos until they reached the blastocyst stage. Whether chromosome preparations are made then is up to the clinic. Knowledge about chromosomal preparations would add to our body of knowledge about the techniques of IVF.

Some clinics do not culture embryos beyond the eight-cell stage. They discard them, or perhaps use them for research, or even for donation to other couples. It is essential to know the limitations of the culture system because one of the fundamental aspects of IVF is that a child might be born from the embryo in culture. Every embryo grown is a potential child to be born nine months later. This is the primary ethical problem we face. That baby must not be put in any jeopardy due to lack of care. It is essential to avoid replacing abnormal embryos if this is possible. It is essential to balance the clinical treatments and the embryology, to ensure that embryonic growth is as satisfactory as possible. Some clinics might proceed without assessing embryonic growth *in vitro*, but their success rate might be low, and many embryos might be abnormal.

References

Angell, R.R., Aitken, R.J., Van Look, P.F.A., Lumsden, M.A., and Templeton, A.A. (1983) Chromosome abnormalities in human embryos after *in vitro* fertilization. *Nature* 303: 336–38

Edmonds, D.K., Lindsay, K.S., Miller, J.F., Williamson, E., and Wood, P.J. (1982) Early embryonic mortality in women. *Fertility and Sterility* 38: 447–53

Leese, H.J. and Barton, A.M. (1984) Pyruvate and glucose uptake by mouse ova and preimplantation embryos. *Journal of Reproduction and Fertility* 72: 9–13

Leese, H.J., Hooper, M.A.K., Edwards, R.G., and Ashwood-Smith, M.J. (1986) Uptake of pyruvate by early human embryos determined by a non-invasive technique. *Human Reproduction* 3: 181–82

FIVE

The use of human pre-embryos for infertility research

P. R. Braude, V. N. Bolton, and M. H. Johnson

The technique of *in vitro* fertilization (IVF) has led to the birth of almost 1000 babies worldwide, alleviating the misery of childlessness for nearly as many couples. The development of this technique has raised many ethical problems, not least the question of whether research using human pre-embryos should be permitted. This chapter considers some of the arguments for continuing research into infertility that involves the use of human pre-embryos derived from fertilization *in vitro*. Four major areas of research are considered: (a) investigation of male infertility; (b) improvement of the low success rate of therapeutic IVF; (c) improvement of cryopreservation techniques; (d) investigation of reasons for early pregnancy loss. In each case, the necessity for studies using human, rather than animal, pre-embryos is explained. It is suggested that society, and medical scientists, must decide whether it is more acceptable to prohibit research using the human pre-embryo, in which case the adult patients become the experimental subjects, or permit such research, subject to careful control and regulation.

Childlessness, as the previous chapters show, affects a significant proportion of the population. The technique of *in vitro* fertiliz-ation (IVF) has done much to alleviate the misery of infertility for many by providing a means of therapy where all conventional forms of treatment had failed, or where none was available previously. In addition to its therapeutic advantages, the fertilization of human egg cells (oocytes) *in vitro* has made it possible to investigate for the first time certain aspects of human reproductive failure.

Male infertility

A major contribution of IVF to the alleviation of reproductive failure has been in the treatment of the clinically infertile male. A man who has been diagnosed as infertile because he has very few spermatozoa (oligozoospermia) can now father his own child by this technique (Cohen *et al.* 1985). Thus clinical infertility associated with an abnormal semen analysis (Mortimer 1985a) or with abnormal functional tests of sperm transport (Mortimer 1985b) is not synonymous with lack of fertilizing capacity. However, conventional measures of semen analysis (count, motility, and morphology) do not yet allow us to predict which semen samples will be able to fertilize oocytes *in vitro*. Although many tests of spermatozoal function are available – such as the postcoital test, the crossed penetration or crossed hostility test (to examine for hostile cervical mucus), sperm retrieval at laparoscopy, and the zona-free hamster oocyte penetration assay (Yanagimachi 1984) – the relationship between these tests and fertility *in vitro* is undefined. Thus, although generalizations about semen quality and fertilizing capacity can be made, based on the statistics from therapeutic IVF programmes (Mahadevan and Trounson 1984), these are of little help in deciding whether an individual man is fertile.

There are two possible approaches to obtaining more reliable prognostic criteria. Where the male partner in an infertile relationship shows a significant abnormality on semen analysis, the couple may be included in a therapeutic IVF programme. If fertilization is successful and is followed by embryo replacement and perhaps a pregnancy, there is no need for further investigation. However, if fertilization fails, it is not immediately obvious whether spermatozoal or oocyte factors are involved. In this procedure, although it is the male partner who is being investigated, it is the female partner who is the experimental subject. She may well have to endure an unnecessary anaesthetic and operation in order to obtain the information that a single semen sample from her partner was, on this occasion, incapable of fertilizing her oocytes.

An alternative and more direct approach to the problem of knowing whether a clinically infertile man can father a child is to use donated human oocytes to try to achieve fertilization *in vitro*, using the abnormal semen sample. Here, the specific objective is to try and define the characteristics of successful fertilization under standardized conditions, so that criteria can be derived for prognosis for men with semen problems. As the oocyte donors are fertile women who have already agreed to an anaesthetic and operation for the purposes of sterilization (Braude *et al.* 1984), no unnecessary operation has to be performed. Moreover, as there is no intention to achieve a pregnancy on this occasion, and as the test can be repeated later with oocytes donated by another woman, there is no pressure to obtain a positive result at the expense of experimental design. As the oocytes or fertilized eggs (pre-embryos) are not destined to be replaced in the woman, the developmental potential of pre-embryos *in vitro* can also be studied – for it is clear that a high proportion of abnormally formed spermatozoa have chromosomal aberrations (Carothers and Beatty 1975) yet can still penetrate oocyte membranes (Cohen 1982). The relevance of semen defects for embryonic failure is undefined but the use of human pre-embryos for research is one way of tackling this problem. For example, it is now possible to prepare, from abnormal semen samples, a population of spermatozoa that are almost exclusively haploid (i.e. have the right number of chromosomes for a sperm cell). If this method is applied to fertilization *in vitro*, it may provide a way of reducing embryo failure caused by chromosome abnormality induced by fertilization with polyploid spermatozoa (i.e. those with too many sets of chromosomes).

When fertilization cannot be achieved *in vitro* because of extremely low spermatozoal numbers or because the spermatozoa show fertilization defects, workers in some laboratories are trying to inject the spermatozoon under the zona pellucida (outer membrane of the egg) or directly into the cytoplasm of the oocyte. Although this technique may be the only hope for some men with severe oligozoospermia, the effects of the technique on the developmental potential of the fertilized oocyte need to be assessed before it is offered as a means of treatment. Obviously, this assessment can only be made if the methods are first perfected on animal oocytes and then tested on human oocytes not destined to be replaced in the uterus.

Improvements to IVF as a therapeutic technique

Although many improvements have been made to the clinical practice of fertilization *in vitro*, and one might now expect a pregnancy rate of 25 per cent per patient per replacement in the best units (Steptoe 1985), the rate of success per pre-embryo is not much more than 10 per cent (Table 5.1). The figure drops to about 8 per cent for ongoing pregnancies per replacement and is even worse per oocyte retrieved.

If we are to improve the success of this technique for the alleviation of infertility we need to understand why almost 90 per cent of pre-embryos fail to implant and why many of those that do implant do not become viable pregnancies. Although epidemiological evidence from therapeutic units indicates the

Table 5.1   Success of pre-embryo replacement

pre-embryos replaced[a]	replacements	pregnancies per replacement (%)	pregnancies per pre-embryo replaced (%)
(A) *From Osborne and Moor (1985)[b]*			
1	377	9.6	9.6
2	328	23.4	13.5
3	190	24.7	9.5
(B) *From Steptoe (1985)[c]*			
1	626	14.6	14.6
2	498	24.8	12.4
3	312	31.4	10.4

[a]Number replaced per replacement procedure.
[b]Reporting figures from Lopata, Craft, Feichtinger, Kerin, Laufer, and Belaisch-Allart.
[c]Bourn Hall, January 1981–December 1983.

direction that experimental investigations should take, and results from animal models help to suggest possible mechanisms for failure, information directly relevant to the human will be obtained only by examining human pre-embryos themselves.

For example, by using donated oocytes fertilized *in vitro* we have found that human pre-embryos can be grown to the four-cell stage with a high degree of success in a wide variety of culture media. However, attempts to culture pre-embryos reliably through to the fully expanded blastocyst stage have met with only limited success (Fig. 5.1). Although the number of pre-embryos examined in our study is small, attempts by large therapeutic units to culture fertilized oocytes through to the fully

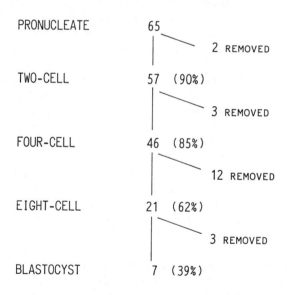

HUMAN EMBRYONIC DEVELOPMENT IN VITRO

PRONUCLEATE 65
2 REMOVED

TWO-CELL 57 (90%)
3 REMOVED

FOUR-CELL 46 (85%)
12 REMOVED

EIGHT-CELL 21 (62%)
3 REMOVED

BLASTOCYST 7 (39%)

Figure 5.1 the development of sixty-five pronucleate pre-embryos derived from fertilization *in vitro* of donated oocytes (Braude *et al.* 1984). Twenty pre-embryos were removed at various developmental stages for biochemical analysis. Percentages refer to the remaining pre-embryos that developed successfully at each stage

expanded blastocyst stage for storage at low temperature (cryo-preservation) yield similar results (Fehilly *et al.* 1985). There is, however, some debate about whether there is a particular stage before blastocyst formation when development of the pre-embryo is most likely to be arrested (Edwards 1985). A number of explanations can be offered for this failure of human pre-embryos to develop *in vitro* to the blastocyst stage. Although poor culture conditions might be responsible, it is difficult to explain why the pre-embryos of one patient stop developing during culture whereas the pre-embryos of another patient form blastocysts in the same culture medium. It is also difficult to explain why some of a cohort of pre-embryos from the same patient form blastocysts but others in the cohort fail. Clearly pre-embryo quality must contribute to the failure.

Research on animal pre-embryos has identified an important event that may explain why a particular stage of development is sensitive. In the mouse, development probably does not depend on gene expression until the two-cell stage (Flach *et al.* 1982). Before this stage normal cellular function, including the first cleavage division, depends on the post-transcriptional products stored in the unfertilized oocyte, that is, on maternally inherited information (Braude *et al.* 1979). If gene activity after the two-cell stage of mouse embryogenesis is prevented experimentally by the use of transcriptional inhibitors, new protein synthesis is prevented and further cleavage of the pre-embryo is blocked (Fig. 5.2). Thus, the inability of the human pre-embryo to activate its genes may be one mechanism by which cleavage of the cells is arrested *in vitro*. Preliminary experiments in our laboratory indicate that the human pre-embryo will cleave from the early two-cell stage to the four-cell stage in the presence of a transcriptional inhibitor. This suggests that both mouse and human pre-embryos may be similarly dependent on maternally inherited information, although the exact stage at which gene activity begins in each species may differ, being the two-cell stage in the mouse and perhaps the four-cell stage in the human. The fact that very few human pre-embryos arrest developmentally before the four-cell stage *in vitro*, together with the significantly higher rate of subsequent attrition of pre-embryos, supports this conclusion. If confirmed, this information will be useful in trying

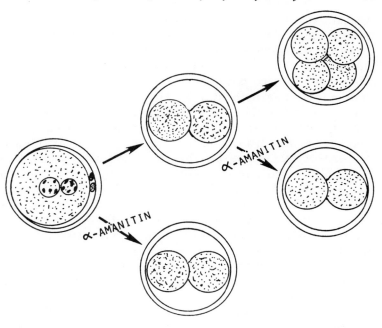

Embryonic Genome Independent   **Embryonic Genome Dependent**
(Stored maternal messenger RNA)   (Embryonic messenger RNA)

Figure 5.2   the developmental potential of mouse pre-embryos cultured in the presence or absence of the transcriptional inhibitor α-amanitin

to determine the factors that may influence or promote gene activity, and so improve the success of development. This phenomenon would not have been detected if research on human pre-embryos was not permitted beyond the mere 'observation' of preimplantation development in culture. Clearly, experiments in which human pre-embryos might be destroyed cannot be justified unless the pre-embryos are created either specifically for research or as 'spares' in therapeutic programmes.

It has been suggested that research which results in the destruction of human pre-embryos is unnecessary and that such work yields no more information than could be gathered from animal experiments alone. However, some data obtained from animal experiments cannot be extrapolated directly to the human, as there are circumstances in which the application of such information may be misleading. For example, sheep oocytes have been removed from their follicles at various times after human chorionic gonadotropin (hCG) has been injected to stimulate their maturation; when these oocytes were cultured *in vitro* until the time at which they would normally have been ovulated, they did not, on fertilization and transfer to recipients, develop normally or produce live young (Trounson, Leeton, and Wood 1982). Extrapolation from these results would suggest that the same might be seen with immature human oocytes cultured *in vitro*. However, Templeton and his colleagues in Edinburgh used donated human oocytes to show that fertilization and cleavage can be obtained in more than half the oocytes removed prematurely from their follicles (Templeton 1985). Even when no hCG at all was given, follicular oocytes were nonetheless fertilized; of the seven cleaving pre-embryos that Templeton obtained two developed *in vitro* to the blastocyst stage. But successful culture *in vitro* even to the blastocyst stage does not imply developmental competence and further investigation is needed to support anecdotal reports of pregnancies by IVF obtained after maturation *in vitro* of 'immature' human oocytes (Veeck *et al.* 1983). This phenomenon cannot be investigated in any controlled way in a therapeutic situation without the chances of pregnancy being jeopardized for the woman from whom the oocytes are obtained. Such experiments should only be performed with oocytes and pre-embryos not destined for replacement or transfer.

Low temperature storage of oocytes and pre-embryos

Low temperature storage (cryostorage) of human pre-embryos is one means by which the clinical success of IVF can be enhanced (Fehilly *et al.* 1985). It is already clear that if pre-embryos surplus to those replaced in the stimulated cycle are frozen, successful pregnancies can be achieved after these pre-embryos have been thawed and replaced in a subsequent cycle. However, although the techniques for freezing human pre-embryos are based on those for cryostorage of animal pre-embryos (Whittingham and

Wood 1984), many human pre-embryos surplus to therapeutic regimes have been destroyed in the attempts to attain a successful pregnancy. Indeed, experts are still uncertain as to the optimum developmental stage for successful cryopreservation and continued development after thawing. This type of research may not be considered by some to constitute experimentation – but it is precisely that, and it represents the only way in which this aspect of IVF technology can progress. The sad fact is that the techniques have had to be developed in a trial-and-error fashion, instead of by systematic research. Once again the infertile woman has been the experimental subject who has had to bear with the good intentions of the clinical scientist trying to perfect techniques using her pre-embryos instead of pre-embryos that were never destined for replacement. Although as a group these patients may be considered to have the most to gain from this work, without adequate preliminary controlled research they also have the most to lose – medically, emotionally, and often financially.

Successful cryostorage of unfertilized oocytes has proved more difficult to achieve than storage of pre-embryos. Indeed, the mouse is the only species in which freshly ovulated oocytes have been preserved successfully and live offspring obtained after fertilization *in vitro*. Even here, there was a significant increase in the incidence of polyploidy in the resulting embryos (Whittingham 1985). If techniques for freezing oocytes are to be developed and new methods such as vitrification (Rall and Fahy 1985) are to be applied to human material, the risks of such procedures must be assessed as fully as possible before they are accepted as a mode of treatment. This will necessarily entail not only attempts to achieve fertilization of oocytes after freezing and thawing but also an evaluation of the chromosome complement and developmental capacity of the resulting pre-embryos. The only safe way of developing these methods, once animal studies are complete, would be to test them first on donated or 'spare' human oocytes.

If it proves possible to mature human oocytes *in vitro* before fertilization, this process, combined with that of cryostorage of oocytes, will become a powerful therapeutic tool. If the stage of maturation that oocytes had reached could be determined non-destructively, perhaps from the follicular fluids or from the mitotic state of the surrounding cumulus cells (Westergaard 1985), it might be possible to complete their maturation *in vitro* either before freezing or after thawing, and to fertilize only as many oocytes as were thought to be necessary to obtain a pregnancy for a particular couple. Hyperstimulation of the ovary and surgical retrieval of oocytes would only be needed once, and a pre-embryo could be replaced as often as necessary to achieve a pregnancy. This technology would also provide a means of helping women who, due to malignant disease, have to have their ovaries removed, or undergo cytotoxic treatment or radiotherapy resulting in sterility, perhaps at a young age. Such women could have their oocytes frozen before therapy, in the same way as men undergoing similar treatment might have their spermatozoa stored.

Early pregnancy loss

Finally, many pregnancies arising from conception *in vivo* and *in vitro* are known to fail at very early stages of gestation. These failures may show up as overt early miscarriages, or perhaps as missed abortions (the finding of an empty gestation sac by ultrasound), or merely as 'biochemical pregnancies' (in which raised levels of hCG are detected in the blood) (Edmonds *et al.* 1982). It is also quite likely that many pregnancies fail even before the products of trophoblast activity are measurable. The exact causes of these early pregnancy losses are unknown, as is the frequency of their occurrence. Some of them may reflect a failure of the totipotential blastomeres of the pre-embryo at the early cleavage stage to differentiate into the trophectoderm and inner cell mass of the blastocyst, for it is the inner cell mass that includes the precursor tissue of the true embryo. Failure of inner cell mass formation can be induced experimentally in animal pre-embryos (Braude *et al.* 1983). The resulting trophoblastic vesicle may resemble a normal blastocyst – for example it may produce trophoblast hormones – but it does not have the potential to form an embryo. The finding that some human blastocysts cultured *in vitro* may lack an inner cell mass (Mohr 1984) adds some credence to this hypothesis about what causes empty gestation sacs and biochemical pregnancies.

Some progress has been made in identifying the mechanisms by which the first differentiative event occurs in the mammalian pre-embryo (Johnson *et al.* 1984), but whether and when similar mechanisms operate in the human pre-embryo is unknown. However, it is the experimental study of these events in the human pre-embryo which may help in our understanding of early pregnancy failure. Although it is too soon to believe that our understanding of the normal mechanisms of differentiation will lead to a means of preventing early pregnancy loss, the ability to explain the origin of these events may provide a small measure of comfort for those who suffer the distressing consequences of miscarriage.

Conclusion

In this chapter we have outlined four very obvious and important areas in which research on human pre-embryos would be of value in diagnosis, prognosis, or therapy for the infertile couple. As medical scientists we can offer only our predictions and assessments.

(1) We would not be asking the questions raised in this symposium if no research had been done on human pre-embryos created for research purposes. After the first successful fertilization *in vitro*, Edwards, Steptoe, and Purdy did not move directly to a therapeutic programme. They first carefully observed pre-embryos growing *in vitro* that were created for that purpose only. Few would now deny the value of this research, nor want its benefits denied to patients. It is important to be sure that the interests of the potential beneficiaries of further research are not overlooked.

(2) Our examples are drawn conservatively. The research that we propose, and the benefits that are likely to result from it, are almost self-evident. However, research involves the unanticipated and the novel. Areas of research that at present seem to be of only marginal clinical value may become compelling as a result of the sort of research proposed above. Moreover, there are undoubtedly other as yet unimagined areas in which research on human pre-embryos will offer clinical advantages. A complete

prohibition on research precludes not only obvious and calculable benefits but also the possibility of unenvisaged future benefits, whereas regulated research would allow any potential benefit to be reassessed in the light of new experience and clinical need.

(3) In essence there is a choice: either the human pre-embryo can be used as the subject of controlled and regulated research, so that the treatment that is applied eventually to the infertile couple has been tried and tested; or the infertile patients, in partnership with their own pre-embryos, can become the joint subjects for research. In both cases research on pre-embryos is occurring, but only in the latter case are adult humans placed in the position of being the subjects of experimentation. The medical scientist needs to know which, if either, of these alternatives is acceptable to society.

Acknowledgements

P.R. Braude and M.H. Johnson are recipients of a Medical Research Council programme grant.

References

Braude, P.R., Pelham, H.R.B., Flach, G., and Lobatto, R. (1979) Post-transcriptional control in the early mouse embryo. *Nature* 282: 102–105

Braude, P.R., Johnson, M.H., Bolton, V.N., and Pratt, H.P.M. (1983) Cleavage and differentiation of the early embryo. In P.G. Crosignani and B.L. Rubin (eds) *In Vitro Fertilization and Embryo Transfer*. London: Academic Press (Serono Clinical Colloquia on Reproduction vol. 4) pp. 211–28

Braude, P.R., Bright, M.V., Douglas, C.P., Milton, P.J., Robinson, R.E., Williamson, J.G., and Hutchison, J. (1984) A regimen for obtaining mature human oocytes from donors for research into human fertilization *in vitro*. *Fertility and Sterility* 42: 34–8

Carothers, A.D. and Beatty, R.A. (1975) The recognition and incidence of haploid and polyploid spermatozoa in man, rabbit and mouse. *Journal of Reproduction and Fertility* 44: 487–500

Cohen, J. (1982) *Interactie Tussen Menselijke Zaadcellen en Hamstereicellen*. Ph.D. Thesis, University of Rotterdam

Cohen, J., Edwards, R.G., Fehilly, C.B., Fishel, S., Hewitt, J., Purdy, J., Rowland, G., Steptoe, P., and Webster, J. (1985) *In vitro* fertilization: a treatment for male infertility. *Fertility and Sterility* 43: 422–32

Edmonds, D.K., Lindsay, K.S., Miller, J.F., Williamson, E., and Wood, P.J. (1982) Early embryonic mortality in women. *Fertility and Sterility* 38: 447–57

Edwards, R.G. (1985) Major problems in IVF. In Thompson *et al.* (1985), pp. 79–92

Fehilly, C.B., Cohen, J., Simons, R.F., Fishel, S.B., and Edwards, R.G. (1985) Cryopreservation of cleaving embryos and expanded blastocysts in the human: a comparative study. *Fertility and Sterility* 44: 638–44

Flach, G., Johnson, M.H., Braude, P.R., Taylor, R.A.S., and Bolton, V.N. (1982) The transition from maternal to embryonic control in the 2-cell mouse embryo. *EMBO (European Molecular Biology Organization) Journal* 1: 681–86

Johnson, M.H., Ziomek, C.A., Reeve, W.J.D., Pratt, H.P.M., Goodall, H., and Handyside, A.H. (1984) The mosaic organization of the preimplantation mouse embryo. In J. Van Blerkom and P. Motta (eds) *Ultrastructure of Reproduction and Early Development*. The Hague: Martinus Nijhoff (Current Topics in Ultrastructure Research) pp. 205–17

Mahadevan, M.M., and Trounson, A.O. (1984) The influence of seminal characteristics on the success rate of human in vitro fertilization. *Fertility and Sterility* 42: 400–405

Mohr, L. (1984) Assessment of human embryos. In A. Trounson and C. Wood (eds) *In Vitro Fertilization and Embryo Transfer*. Edinburgh: Churchill Livingstone

Mortimer, D. (1985a) The male factor in infertility, part I: semen analysis. *Current Problems in Obstetrics, Gynaecology and Fertility* 8 (7): 1–87

Mortimer, D. (1985b) The male factor in infertility, part II: sperm function testing. *Current Problems in Obstetrics, Gynaecology and Fertility* 8 (8): 1–75

Osborne, J.C. and Moor, R.M. (1985) Oocyte maturation and developmental competence. In Thompson *et al.* (1985) pp. 101–14

Rall, W.F. and Fahy, G.M. (1985) Ice-free cryopreservation of mouse embryos at −196°C by vitrification. *Nature* 313: 573–75

Steptoe, P.C. (1985) Studies in pregnancy established by *in vitro* fertilisation. In Thompson *et al.* (1985) pp. 241–51

Templeton, A.A. (1985) Ovulation timing and IVF. In Thompson *et al.* (1985) pp. 45–59

Thompson, W., Joyce, D., and Newton, J.R. (eds) (1985) *In Vitro Fertilisation and Donor Insemination.* London: Royal College of Obstetricians and Gynaecologists (Proceedings of 12th Study Group, 1984)

Trounson, A., Leeton, J.F., and Wood, C. (1982) *In vitro* fertilization and embryo transfer in the human. In R. Rolland, E.V. Van Hall, S.G. Hillier, K.P. McNatty and J. Schoemaker (eds) *Follicular Maturation and Ovulation.* Amsterdam: Elsevier, pp. 313–25

Veeck, L.L., Wortham, J.W., Jr, Witmyer, J., Sandow, B.A., Acosta, A.A., Garcia, J.E., Jones, G.S., and Jones, H.W., Jr (1983) Maturation and fertilization of morphologically immature human oocytes in a program of *in vitro* fertilization. *Fertility and Sterility* 39: 594–602

Westergaard, L. (1985) Follicular atresia in relation to oocyte morphology in non-pregnant and pregnant women. *Journal of Reproduction and Fertility* 74: 113–18

Whittingham, D.G. (1985) Human oocyte and embryo freezing. In Thompson *et al.* (1985) pp. 269–74

Whittingham, D.G. and Wood, M. (1984) Low temperature storage of mammalian embryos. *Bibliography of Reproduction* 43 (5): A1–A12

Yanagimachi, R. (1984) Zona-free hamster eggs: their use in assessing fertilizing capacity and examining chromosomes of human spermatozoa. *Gamete Research* 10: 187–232

Discussion

Jacobs: It is very easy to get spare eggs. We can go further these days and say that it is very easy to get spare eggs from follicles with a defined endocrine milieu. Endocrinologists can now match the intrafollicular fluid concentration of hormones closely to what embryologists tell us they think it should be. We can use an analogue of luteinizing hormone releasing hormone (LHRH) to desensitize the pituitary and thereby prevent the patients from secreting their own gonadotropins. We can then give a gonadotropin preparation containing either equal amounts of luteinizing hormone (LH) and follicle-stimulating hormone (FSH) or FSH alone. After this method of ovarian stimulation the patient goes through the usual procedure of *in vitro* fertilization. In work done in collaboration with Richard Porter and Ian Craft, we found that the number of oocytes and cleaving embryos was the same with either LH plus FSH or with FSH alone.

A lot of our patients who came for *in vitro* fertilization had polycystic ovaries, a condition that is easy to diagnose on an ultrasound scan. After the treatment I have just described, these patients produce about twice as many eggs, on average, as those without polycystic ovaries – often more than twenty eggs per stimulated cycle. The concentration of testosterone in the follicular fluid was higher in fluids obtained from polycystic ovaries, and was higher when ovulation was stimulated by FSH plus LH rather than FSH alone. Adjusting the gonadotropic stimulation of the ovary therefore provides large numbers of eggs from a preoperatively definable endocrine milieu.

Modell: Your point was that if research is to be limited to women who are being treated for infertility, they will be exposed to more invasive investigations than would otherwise be needed, wasn't it, Dr Braude?

Braude: Not necessarily, although this may be the case where IVF is being attempted with severely suboptimal sperm. If, by research using human oocytes, we could establish reliable parameters for predicting the absence or presence of fertilizing potential, unnecessary operations would be minimized.

Modell: I thought there was a specific objection to creating pre-embryos for research.

Braude: That is a separate issue. It seems to me that if people object to research on human pre-embryos on moral grounds, they must object to research on pre-embryos regardless of their origin, for in moral terms it cannot make any difference whether the pre-embryo happens to be generated as a result of research or is surplus to a therapeutic programme. In both cases research is being done on a human pre-embryo. Any attempt to separate these two seems artificial. Presumably, if they are to be consistent, those people also object to the very research that has led to the success of IVF for the infertile couple.

Modell: I thought you made the point that if research was limited to a couple seeking treatment for infertility you would have to get the ovum from the woman. This would involve her in anaesthesia and other clinical investigations that she would not otherwise have to undergo. That is an important issue. In fact, similar things have already happened in the past. For instance, when the obstetric techniques for antenatal diagnosis of the haemoglobino-pathies were being developed, many states in the USA specifically forbade research on human embryonic material of any kind. Therefore these techniques were developed elsewhere.

Braude: That is a very good point. In this country those techniques were developed on patients destined for abortion.

Modell: One effect in the USA was that women who were at high risk of having a seriously ill infant, and needed these diagnostic procedures because they desperately wanted a normal child, had to have the new techniques developed on them. Some of them lost much-wanted babies because the techniques could not be developed on pregnant women attending for abortion. Some of these decisions include irrational elements that can have disastrous consequences for patients.

Edwards: We have never established research embryos but have always used the spares from an IVF programme. It is possible to argue that this was not so when we started work in Oldham – that the embryos I showed were research embryos. My weak defence has always been that these studies were necessary because it was essential to test some for normality before any could be replaced in the mother. We could not risk abnormal babies. The embryos we now use for research have three pronuclei or abnormal cleavage. These have given us certain pieces of valuable information. We are using embryos that could not be replaced in the mother and we call this 'abortion *in vitro*'. This is very similar to the use of aborted material for research in other areas, such as making vaccines. It comes under the laws about using aborted foetuses for research.

We did not establish research embryos after those early days because we felt this would open the door to the use of thousands of embryos for research. Moreover, our method gives the embryo a certain status because all normal embryos are replaced or frozen for later replacement. The abnormal embryo is used for research but no others; there is no intention to replace them, and there cannot be such an intent. We felt that the decision about providing embryos purely for research should be taken by a higher authority than the scientists and medical doctors who are involved in *in vitro* fertilization.

McLaren: It seems very difficult to devise means of assessing normality in human pre-embryos if you only allow yourself to look at the abnormal ones.

Edwards: The nuclei are abnormal in chromosome numbers but the embryos are metabolically normal. These embryos give us a great deal of information.

Johnson: It is very important to emphasize that when we are developing a new technology we are doing research. We are fooling ourselves if we believe that research on spare pre-embryos from a therapeutic programme is different from research on pre-embryos created for the purpose. Although Bob Edwards says he doesn't create pre-embryos for research purposes, that is exactly what happened during the development of IVF technology. He and Patrick Steptoe said they would not put pre-embryos produced by IVF back into women until they were confident of the normality of the pre-embryos. That means creating pre-embryos for research. If it is legitimate to undertake research on spare pre-embryos because one's *intention* ultimately is therapeutic, then it must also be legitimate to *create* pre-embryos if one's intention ultimately is therapeutic. It is the question of intent that is paramount.

The true alternatives are either to permit regulated and approved research (in which case the source of the pre-embryos ceases to be material) or to stop it. This choice is the only real one, and the latter option is only rarely discussed. We could as a society decide that infertility was a condition to accept and live with, just as we do with many other conditions. Our efforts could then go into counselling and changing social priorities. But if infertility is to be cured rather than accepted, the research required will inevitably involve use of pre-embryos, and their source is immaterial, since the motivation is the same regardless.

Baird: You and Peter Braude have pointed out that research is an integral part of the development of new treatment. Using hyperstimulation to produce many eggs is not ideal, in that the chance that any one of the resulting embryos will have the full developmental competence to go on and form a baby is about 10 per cent. To investigate a better means of inducing hyperstimulation, one can set up a randomized trial comparing one method of stimulation with another method. But the very nature of that trial means that if one treatment is better than another, one is compromising the full potential of at least half the embryos that are produced, because they are not getting the optimum stimulation. It would be impossible to conduct any form of clinical treatment without in some way experimenting to the detriment of a particular group of embryos.

Rodeck: Twenty per cent of Peter Braude's pre-embryos went up to the blastocyst stage. What is the longest tme they can be kept in culture?

Edwards: The longest survival has been until day nine, and this was then fixed for electron microscopy. The outgrowths of tissues can of course be kept for longer than that.

Rodeck: What proportion go up to day nine?

Edwards: Very few.

McLaren: The length of time a pre-embryo can be kept in culture and the developmental stage to which it will develop in culture are quite different. Blastocysts kept for nine days in culture are unlikely to have reached a stage equivalent to that reached by a nine-day embryo *in vivo*.

Edwards: The one examined at day nine had the endoderm migrating round the blastocystic cavity. Another attached to the plastic vessel at day nine and formed tissues. They are probably equivalent to a seven-day or eight-day embryo, although there is no definite knowledge of growth *in vivo* at these stages.

Clothier: Professor Dunstan, is there any philosophical difference between spare embryos and those created for research?

Dunstan: I personally would not maintain that there is a morally significant difference between those two but I think Professor Dyson believes there is.

Dyson: In ethics one is concerned with intention, with the nature of an act, and with its consequences. Clearly, using an embryo which is already being produced with a therapeutic intention could be argued to be different from creating one for specific research purposes. There are analogies to this. For some transplants we use organs which are a by-product of other interventions rather than taking them directly from living human beings. There are distinctions there.

Braude: What about the mother who makes a deliberate decision to give one of her functioning kidneys to her child?

Dyson: The main argument in ethics would be that the importance of intention, though intangible, can be underestimated. That intentions can affect the general moral quality of society has to be borne in mind when this sort of question is asked. Therefore using an embryo acquired as a result of therapeutic purposes is a different matter from manufacturing it deliberately for research.

At the beginning of your paper, Dr Braude, you spoke about different kinds of research and you seemed to me to be levelling down different types or intentions of research to one kind. This is something which we might have to look at carefully. In other aspects of medicine we draw distinctions between different kinds of research in relation to different kinds of patients. For adult human beings there are certain limits and for children there are different limits. Are you saying that you don't like those distinctions at all in relation to research or that they don't apply to the pre-embryo but do apply to other human beings? Are you therefore making an assumption about the ontological difference between pre-embryos and other beings?

Braude: The question of the moral status of embryos was raised many times in the Warnock Report (Warnock 1984). It is impossible for any of us to say that a specific early pre-embryo is destined to become a child. The four-cell or eight-cell pre-embryos that I might have for research may have become a hydatidiform mole or a teratocarcinoma, or they may have aborted. I therefore do not believe that they have the same moral status as a child. Moral status to my mind develops with time. As you have said, the moral status of a child is different to that of an adult. For society to say that they are the same is the easy way out. The time has come for us to confront this question.

Clothier: We must return to that topic later.

Edwards: We should also find time to discuss the ethics of freezing embryos, which is related to their moral status and rights.

Reference

Warnock, M. (Chairman) (1984) *Report of the Committee of Inquiry into Human Fertilisation and Embryology.* London: HMSO (Department of Health & Social Security) Cmnd. 9314

SIX

Analysis of foetal DNA for the diagnosis and management of genetic disease

D.J. Weatherall, J.B. Clegg, D.R. Higgs, J.M. Old, J.S. Wainscoat, S.L. Thein, and W.G. Wood

The new techniques of recombinant DNA technology are making it possible to find the molecular defect of many single-gene disorders and to study at least some of the complex genetic interactions which underlie a number of common conditions such as diabetes and coronary artery disease. In the long term these techniques may lead to a better understanding of early human development and hence the cause of congenital malformation. These methods have already been applied to the early prenatal diagnosis of single-gene disorders. Provided that the current techniques of foetal DNA sampling turn out to be safe, research on early human embryos directed towards the diagnosis of genetic disease will have a low priority in the immediate future. Animal models are also likely to be the major source of information about developmental genetics over the next few years. However, as more is learnt about the genetic regulation of development, the time will come when work on earlier stages of human development may provide valuable information about the prevention and treatment of genetic disease and congenital malformation.

If we are to assess the scientific and medical potential of research on embryos we need to define what the tools of molecular biology have told us already about genetic disease and how far current technology is likely to take us in the future. Are there particular areas of investigation of the human genome in general, and of developmental genetics in particular, which can only be explored further by work on human embryos? Here we shall try to summarize what is known about the molecular defects of genetic disease and highlight those areas in which valuable information might be obtained from studies of the earlier stages of human development.

The spectrum of genetic disease and congenital malformation

About 1 per cent of infants are born with a genetic defect or congenital anomaly. Genetic diseases account for an important fraction of admissions of children to hospital and of deaths under the age of fifteen years in developed countries (Weatherall 1985). Genetic diseases are divided into single-gene disorders which may have a dominant, recessive or X-linked form of inheritance, and chromosomal abnormalities. In addition, at least some congenital malformations have a strong genetic component, and genetic factors play an important role in many of the common disorders of adult life, such as diabetes mellitus, epilepsy, psychoses, and autoimmune and premature vascular disease, although environmental factors are also among the causes of these conditions. Although the common cancers are not inherited, malignant transformation leads to fundamental changes in the genetic machinery of cells, changes which are handed on to the progeny of those cells.

The total impact of genetic disease on society is discussed in detail elsewhere (Weatherall 1985). Genetic factors contribute significantly to mortality and morbidity in the developed countries and, as social conditions improve and the rates for early neonatal and infant deaths from malnutrition and infection are reduced, they will pose an equally serious problem in the developing countries.

Methods for studying human molecular defects

Several accounts of the methods of DNA analysis, directed at non-specialist readers, have been published recently (Emery 1984; Weatherall 1985). It is now possible to identify and isolate human genes by the use of probes which find their partners by molecular hybridization – a process in which two complementary strands of DNA associate with each other. Messenger RNA can be isolated from cells in which its parent gene is expressed and used as a template, or blueprint, to make complementary DNA (cDNA). If the latter is radioactively labelled, it can be used as a probe to search the genome for its DNA counterpart. A family of bacterial enzymes called restriction endonucleases have been discovered which cut DNA at predictable sites. Fragments of total human DNA digests produced by these enzymes can be inserted into plasmids or bacteriophages which replicate in bacteria. In this way 'libraries' containing most of the human genome can be grown in bacterial cells. Methods have been developed to identify individual genes in bacterial cells which can then be grown so that the gene can be obtained in sufficient quantities to be sequenced or used to make a gene probe. A start has been made on developing systems for analysing the expression of both normal and mutant human genes in the test tube. Finally, a rapid method for analysing human genes, called gene mapping, has been worked out. This entails cutting DNA into small fragments with restriction enzymes, separating them in gels according to their size, blotting the DNA onto filters, and determining the position of a particular gene or gene fragment by hybridization with radioactively labelled probes. The latter will only bind to DNA with an identical, or almost identical, sequence.

If the biochemical basis for a genetic disease is known it is usually possible to isolate the offending gene. For example, if the disorder is due to an enzyme deficiency a gene probe can be made, based on the protein sequence of the enzyme, and used to search a gene library for its partner. In this way the mutant gene can be isolated and sequenced. Furthermore, one of the particular advantages of these new techniques is that it is possible to 'find' genes for disorders in which the underlying abnormality is completely unknown. The idea is as follows. Restriction enzymes cut DNA at specific sequences. Every few hundred bases in human DNA there are sequences that vary in their susceptibility to cleavage with a particular enzyme. This harmless genetic variability results in 'restriction fragment length polymorphisms' (RFLPs) – inherited differences in the length of DNA fragments generated with restriction enzymes. Strictly speaking these sites are dimorphisms: the sequence is either identified by an enzyme or it is not. However, there are other forms of RFLP which are turning out to be particularly useful for gene hunting. So-called hypervariable regions generate fragments of different sizes when they are cut with restriction enzymes; these length variations are inherited. These regions, which consist of repetitive sequences (satellite DNA), provide a particularly useful source of genetic markers (Jeffreys *et al*. 1985). Thus if we wish to find a gene for a disease of unknown cause, we study a family to see if an RFLP linkage can be established. If we find a linkage it is then possible, by various tricks of genetic engineering, to work along a chromosome towards the putative locus for the disorder.

These techniques are revolutionizing human genetics. In the sections that follow I shall cite a few examples of what they have told us so far about human molecular defects.

Human molecular defects

Genes control the structure of peptide chains – long strings of amino acids which are the basic building blocks of enzymes and other important proteins. The information which determines the order of amino acids in a protein is held in the DNA of its individual gene by virtue of the particular order of its constituent bases, the DNA being made up of four nucleotide bases: adenine, guanine, cytosine, and thymine. This information is transferred from the nucleus of cells to their cytoplasm, where protein synthesis takes place by means of an intermediary called messenger RNA. This is a mirror image of the gene from which it is copied, or transcribed. Thus when a gene is to be transcribed a messenger RNA copy is made from DNA and, after processing, is transported to the cytoplasm where it acts as a template for a complex process whereby amino acids are added one by one in the appropriate order until a peptide chain is synthesized. Thus the flow of genetic information in cells can be represented as DNA→RNA→protein. The way in which this system is controlled is not yet understood but the most important factor seems to be the rate at which the gene is transcribed; there is some fine adjustment at the translational level.

Molecular defects of single-gene disorders

Recent studies of the thalassaemias, genetic anaemias, and the commonest genetic diseases, have told us in detail how a single base change (mutation) in a gene can profoundly modify its function (Orkin *et al.* 1983; Collins and Weissman 1984; Weatherall and Wainscoat 1985). The mutation may produce a premature stop codon, so that when messenger RNA is translated, shortened, and therefore functionally useless, peptide chains are produced. Because amino acids are encoded by a triplet code, loss or insertion of one, two, or four bases in a gene throws the reading frame out of sequence. Most genes have their coding regions (exons) divided into several pieces by lengths of DNA of unknown function called introns. Since primary RNA transcripts contain both intron and exon sequences the introns have to be cut out and the exons precisely spliced together before messenger RNAs move into the cell cytoplasm to act as templates for protein synthesis. Several types of thalassaemia result from mutations which interfere with splicing. For example, single base changes at the junctions between introns and exons may prevent splicing; no normal messenger RNA is produced. Even more surprisingly, base changes within introns or exons can produce alternative splice sites which result in the production of both normal and abnormally spliced messenger RNA; the latter cannot be used as a template for protein synthesis. All mammalian genes have sequences in common at their 5' flanking regions which play a critical role in the regulation of transcription. Single base changes in these regions can reduce their rate of transcription, hence the output of the product of the gene is also reduced. In addition to these subtle mutations some forms of thalassaemia result from deletions which remove part or all of the globin genes, or from inversions or other major rearrangements of the globin gene clusters.

It seems likely, therefore, that we already have a reasonable idea of the repertoire of the molecular mechanisms that can give rise to single-gene disorders. Recent studies of the mutant genes of patients with Christmas disease, haemophilia, growth hormone deficiency, antithrombin III deficiency, and low density lipoprotein receptor deficiency support this prediction (reviewed by Weatherall 1985). Because the biochemical basis for these conditions was known it was relatively easy to make gene probes to isolate the mutant genes. However, spectacular progress has also been made in defining the genes for disorders in which the cause is completely unknown. For example, using RFLP linkage analysis it has been possible to obtain linkages for Huntington's chorea (Gusella *et al.* 1983), Duchenne muscular dystrophy (reviewed by Davies 1985), and, very recently, polycystic disease of the kidney (Reeders *et al.* 1985) and cystic fibrosis (reviewed by de la Chapelle 1985). Over the next few years it should be possible to define these loci more closely and, ultimately, to identify their gene products and hence the molecular basis for these common conditions.

Polygenic diseases

The molecular analysis of polygenic diseases, common diseases in which it is thought that several genes and the action of environmental factors are implicated, is much more complex than that of single-gene disorders, mainly because in most cases it is still not clear which genes are involved and to what extent inheritance, compared with environment, is responsible for their causation.

Diabetes and autoimmune disease. Genetic factors play an important role in diabetes. For example, individuals who inherit either HLA–B8–DR3, or HLA–B15–DR4 haplotypes have an increased risk of developing type I diabetes. In addition, it is suspected that this kind of diabetes can be precipitated by infection, probably viral; the HLA–DR molecules are important regulators of the immune response. There has been rapid progress in determining the structure of the major histocompatibility genes and many RFLPs have been defined in this large gene complex. By using RFLPs it should be possible to dissect the genetics of the HLA-associated diseases in much greater detail. Similarly, recent work on the T cell receptor and the mechanisms of the interaction of T cells with B cells or other cells provides us with an approach to the molecular analysis of autoimmune disease.

Cardiovascular disease. Very little is known about the pathogenesis of premature vascular disease except that environmental factors such as smoking play a major role. However, a start has been made in analysing what are called 'candidate genes', in this case genes for proteins which may have some relevance to the pathophysiology of vessel wall and lipid metabolism. For example, a number of apolipoprotein genes have been cloned and RFLPs have been defined. It appears that particular polymorphisms are associated with premature vascular disease or abnormalities of lipid metabolism (Karanthansis *et al.* 1983a, b, Rees *et al.* 1983). Progress has also been made in analysing the molecular basis for familial hypercholesterolaemia (high levels of cholesterol in the blood), a condition which results from a deficiency of the low density lipoprotein receptor and which is a common cause of premature coronary artery disease. The gene for the receptor has been cloned and sequenced and it turns out that at least one type of familial hypercholesterolaemia results from a partial deletion (Sudhoff *et al.* 1985). Furthermore, an RFLP has been defined by use of the gene for the low density lipoprotein receptor. About 30 per cent of individuals are heterozygous for this polymorphism, hence it is potentially informative in the early diagnosis of familial hypercholesterolaemia (Humphries *et al.* 1985).

Cancer. In malignant transformation the interactions between environment and genome are even more complex than they are in cardiovascular disease. Familial cancers are rare but neoplasia involves fundamental alterations in the genome of individual cells – changes which are then passed on to the progeny of those cells. Recent work on oncogenes has made it possible to bring together several long-standing observations about the epidemiology and cytogenetics of cancer.

Cellular oncogenes (c-*onc*) seem to be part of the normal genetic machinery of a cell responsible for the control of proliferation, differentiation, and development (Bishop 1985). There is increasing evidence for changes in oncogene activity in different human cancers, although it is still far from clear whether this is the primary cause of malignant transformation. In some cases there is a structural change in an oncogene while in others the chromosomal location of oncogenes may be changed by a translocation which is specific for a particular type of tumour. Examples include the involvement of the c–*abl* oncogene in the translocation which gives rise to the Philadelphia chromosome of chronic myeloid leukaemia, and the involvement of the c–*myc* gene in the different translocations which are found in Burkitt's lymphoma. Indeed, as cytogenetic techniques improve it is apparent that many tumours are associated with specific chromosomal translocations. Equally interesting is the observation that some childhood cancers, for example retinoblastoma (eye tumours) and Wilm's tumour (a common kidney tumour of early life), are associated with mutations or deletions of specific gene loci. If we remain heterozygous for such mutations we may go through life never knowing we have them; the presence of a normal partner (allele) appears to be sufficient to maintain a normal phenotype. On the other hand, if a gene rearrangement in a particular tissue results in homozygosity, malignant transformation will follow (Cavanee *et al.* 1983).

Another novel development in cancer genetics comes from recent studies of the complex gene system involved in regulating the cytochrome *P*-450s (reviewed by Marx 1985a), the haem-containing enzyme system that plays an important role in detoxification. One of the substances which induces activity of enzymes in this gene family is dioxin, which is known to interact with other chemicals to produce malignant changes in experimental animals. The particularly inducible *P*-450 gene codes for the enzyme aryl-hydrocarbon (benzo[α]pyrene) hydroxalase. It has been known for some time that individuals who produce large amounts of this enzyme in response to chemicals are at an increased risk of developing lung cancers; the risk is particularly great for smokers. It now appears that inducibility of this enzyme system shows genetic variability. Hence we have another important approach to studying individual genetic susceptibility to agents which may induce cancer.

Diseases of the nervous system and mental retardation

Recombinant DNA technology has also led to much progress in defining the genetic factors involved in certain chronic neurological disorders and mental retardation. As mentioned earlier (p. 88), an RFLP linkage has been established for Huntington's chorea, despite the fact that the cause of this condition is still completely unknown (Gusella *et al.* 1983). Much progress has been made in defining the chromosomal location and in obtaining linkage markers for Duchenne muscular dystrophy and other X-linked dystrophies and some forms of mental retardation (Davies 1985). It is likely that defining the location of single-gene disorders of this type will ultimately lead to the characterization of the gene loci involved and hence to an understanding of their molecular defects.

The application of recombinant DNA technology is also starting to provide some insights into the complexity of the genetic organization of the central nervous system. Comparison of messenger RNAs from rat brain with those of other tissues suggests that there may be as many as 30 000 neuronal genes, some of which are being isolated and their products analysed (Sutcliffe *et al.* 1984). Progress has also been made in cloning and sequencing DNA from genes for various channels, proteins responsible for the brain's electrical activity. Genes for the subunits of the acetylcholine receptor (an important transmitter molecule in the nervous system) have been sequenced, as has the gene for the sodium channel. Once we can start to understand the regulation of neurotransmitters and their receptors we should be in a better position to work out the molecular defects of a number of intractable neurological and psychiatric disorders. Finally, the recent isolation of the gene for myelin proteins, which is on the X chromosome, promises to provide insight into other serious inherited disorders of the nervous system.

Differentiation, development, and congenital malformation

The most challenging question in human biology, and one of major importance for understanding disorders of development, is how a single fertilized egg with its 10^9 base pairs of DNA turns into a human being. Although there are several well characterized families of human genes which undergo differential expression during development – the globin and muscle protein genes, for example – it seems likely that the more fundamental mechanisms of developmental genetics will have to be worked out in simpler organisms, such as *Drosophila*. However, this information should have relevance to human development. The principles which govern the developmental regulation of gene expression in lower organisms have probably been used, albeit in a modified form, throughout evolution. In this context recent work on *Drosophila* is of particular interest. The homeotic genes, which regulate the development of body segments, have DNA sequences in common with many other species, including man (Gehring 1985). Homeotic mutations in insects result in major developmental abnormalities, including the substitution of one or more segments normally found elsewhere along the body axis.

Another approach which is providing valuable information about developmental genetics is the study of 'foreign' genes that have been injected into fertilized eggs and followed through several generations (reviewed by Palmiter and Brinster 1985). This model is providing valuable information about the physiological consequences of foreign gene expression but, even more importantly, is starting to yield some clues about the molecular mechanisms of foetal abnormality. For example, the insertion of viruses into early embryos produces a variety of defects; a particular abnormality which has been analysed in detail is the one that causes the death of embryos at about the twelfth day of gestation, which appears to be due to the integration of a viral genome into a collagen gene. An even more intriguing example is the observation that animals which have had a particular oncogene inserted into their genomes produce offspring with deformities of their limbs. It turns out that there is a limb deformity gene in mice on chromosome 2 and that the oncogene insert in the transgenic mice with similar deformities is very close to this locus. This type of experiment should make it possible to isolate DNA fragments from segments flanking the oncogene inserts and determine their nucleotide sequences (reviewed by Marx 1985b).

Another important advance in developmental genetics is the

isolation of genes for proteins which are involved in the regulation of growth and differentiation. As well as more general regulatory molecules such as the insulin-like growth factors there are many proteins which take part in the differentiation of specific tissues. For example, a number of proteins of this type play a role in the complex programme in which blood stem cells divide and give rise to progeny which mature into specific types of blood cells (reviewed by Weatherall 1985). Hitherto it has been impossible to isolate and purify these proteins and their receptors, hence it has been difficult to study their activities *in vitro*. Very recently a number of these genes have been isolated, including those for colony-stimulating factor, an important regulator of white cell production, and erythropoietin, the main regulator of the later stages of red cell maturation. Progress has been equally rapid in isolating genes for important mediators of immune responses, for example macrophage-activating factor, the inter-leukins, and tumour necrosis factor. Further work along these lines should provide us with pure proteins with which to study cellular differentiation and investigate disorders resulting from quantitative or qualitative abnormalities of these regulatory molecules.

Chromosome abnormalities underlie many forms of defective development. Restriction enzyme analysis may allow us to identify structural changes of chromosomes which cannot be diagnosed by standard cytogenetic techniques – submicroscopic deletions or insertions, for example. Furthermore, the identification of loci for single-gene disorders associated with major developmental changes may help us to understand the pathophysiology of these conditions (Latt *et al.* 1984).

Practical applications

Prenatal diagnosis

We already have enough experience of the application of DNA analysis to the prenatal diagnosis of single-gene disorders to be sure that this approach is feasible. However, a number of questions remain about the source and the most convenient and economical approaches for analysis of foetal DNA.

Foetal DNA can be obtained either from amniotic fluid cells

or by chorionic villus sampling. The latter entails obtaining a small piece of the chorionic villus tissue which surrounds and nourishes the foetus early in pregnancy and has foetal rather than maternal DNA. The main problem with amniocentesis is that it is usually impossible to obtain enough DNA without growing the amniotic cells in culture for several weeks. Since amniocentesis cannot be performed until about fourteen weeks of gestation this means a long wait for the mother and, if indicated, a late and sometimes difficult termination of pregnancy. On the other hand, chorionic villus sampling can be performed as early as nine weeks and usually yields 20 to 100 μg of DNA. The rate of foetal loss after this procedure is still uncertain; current figures suggest about 4 per cent. It is not yet known whether this procedure results in long-term deleterious effects on the foetus.

Given an adequate supply of foetal DNA several approaches can be used to identify genetic disease (reviewed by Weatherall 1985). Chromosome analysis is very simple and several types of enzyme deficiency can be identified by chemical analysis after cell culture. A number of methods are available for identifying single-gene disorders by DNA analysis. If the molecular defect in a particular disease is known it is sometimes possible to identify the lesion directly, using restriction enzymes. For example the base change which gives rise to the sickle cell mutation can be identified directly by a particular enzyme, and there are several forms of thalassaemia due to point mutations which alter restriction enzyme sites and hence are amenable to the same approach. Disorders which result from gene deletions (loss of all or part of a gene) or rearrangements can also be identified directly by gene mapping. However, this is not feasible for the bulk of single-gene disorders and it is usually necessary to establish an RFLP linkage to the disease by a family study. An attempt is made to identify the parental chromosomes that carry the mutant gene and then to determine whether the foetus has inherited them. The great advantage of this approach is that we need only find a linked RFLP to diagnose the disease; it is not necessary to know anything about the molecular defect. This approach has been used successfully for the prenatal diagnosis of the haemoglobin disorders, haemophilia, muscular dystrophy, and ornithine trans-carbamylase deficiency. Finally, if the molecular pathology is known it is sometimes possible to construct a short gene probe, or oligonucleotide probe, which will identify a single base change directly (Weatherall *et al.* 1985).

Thus, if chorionic villus sampling is found to be associated with an acceptably low rate of foetal loss and does not cause any long-term developmental abnormalities, it will clearly become widely used for prenatal diagnosis. Over the next few years it should be possible to obtain linkage markers for most of the common single-gene disorders and, in the long term, to determine their molecular pathology. The development of prenatal diagnosis programmes will not be without difficulties, however. It is already clear that most single-gene disorders will be heterogeneous at the molecular level and, at least among the X-linked disorders, a high proportion will be due to new mutations. Thus direct gene analysis or RFLP linkage studies may not always allow us to make a diagnosis and we shall have to continue to develop simpler biochemical or immunological methods for identifying genetic diseases.

Gene therapy

There is much interest in the possibility of replacing defective genes. Although it was originally thought that the globin genes might be the prime candidates for the first attempts at gene therapy it is now believed that their complex regulation and the high level of expression required may pose particular difficulties for gene transfer. Thus current activities are directed to replacing genes for enzymes that need to be expressed at a relatively low level in a simple 'always-on' type of regulation (Anderson 1984). There are three candidates: hypoxanthine–guanine phosphori-bosyl transferase, the enzyme which is deficient in the Lesch–Nyhan syndrome; purine nucleoside phosphorylase, the absence of which causes severe immunodeficiency; and adenosine deaminase, the level of which is reduced in children with combined immunodeficiency disease.

There are several approaches to gene transfer, none entirely satisfactory. Direct transfection of DNA into cells is feasible but very inefficient. For this reason attention has turned to the use of delivery systems. A variety of ingenious constructions involving retroviruses have been made and have been used to transfer genes into murine bone marrow cells in culture (Williams *et al.* 1984).

The genetically altered marrow has been implanted into recipient animals and it has been shown that the 'foreign' genes are expressed in the appropriate cells, albeit at a low level. The most recent approach to gene transfer has been the insertion of DNA sequences by homologous recombination, a method which has been used successfully in yeast genetics for some time but which has only recently been applied to human DNA (Smithies *et al.* 1985). This way of inserting foreign genes has the great advantage that it involves site-directed insertion of DNA whereas the other techniques produce random integration of foreign genes into the recipient genome. It seems likely that the most practical approach to gene therapy in the immediate future will be through retrovirus vectors, although a considerable amount of work has to be done to improve the efficiency of this approach and, most importantly, to assess its safety.

All the methods of gene therapy discussed so far are examples of somatic cell gene transfer. However, it is also possible to transfer genes into fertilized mouse eggs. In this case there is the potential for the foreign genes to be integrated into germ-line cells and hence passed on to future generations. Indeed, the transgenic mouse model is proving extremely valuable for studying the factors which are involved in the regulation of foreign genes (Palmiter and Brinster 1985). For example, this technique has been used partially to correct a defect in growth hormone production in mice.

Research on transgenic mice is extremely active. In particular, the factors involved in tissue and developmental specificity of foreign genes inserted into fertilized mouse eggs are being determined; it is likely that this model will provide valuable information about the factors involved in the appropriate functioning of genes in a new environment.

Embryo research and human genetics

It is clear from the preceding sections that rapid progress is being made in working out the molecular pathology of single-gene disorders and that valuable information is also being obtained, albeit more slowly, about the genetic components of polygenic diseases. Chorionic villus sampling provides an immensely

powerful approach for developing prenatal diagnosis programmes for the common single-gene disorders. Gene therapy
will undoubtedly be developed over the next few years although
it may well be a long time before it is applicable to more than a
handful of single-gene disorders. Thus the scene is set for major
advances in the prevention and treatment of genetic diseases. Do
we need to change our focus of research from chorionic tissue to
early embryos?

The notion that it might be possible to 'biopsy' fertilized eggs,
identify those that carry defective genes, and replant those which
do not, is attractive. However, it would require a major scaling-
down of our diagnostic procedures. Furthermore, it is not known
whether the very early human conceptus would be amenable to
this type of interference. In any case, we doubt if there is any
reason to pursue this line of research in the immediate future
provided that chorionic villus sampling turns out to be safe and
reliable for prenatal diagnosis. The technique of chorionic villus
sampling causes less inconvenience to the mother than attempts to
remove eggs for *in vitro* fertilization.

Probably the most important area for future research, and one
which undoubtedly will require human embryonic material, is
developmental genetics. Although this field of study will probably confine itself to animal models for the foreseeable future, a
time must come when embryo research will provide valuable
information about the genetic regulation of the very early stages
of development and, even more importantly, the molecular
pathology of early human embryos. But, again, this work is
unlikely to have high priority in the immediate future. Since so
little is known about developmental genetics it would be
extremely difficult to know what questions to ask; there is a great
deal of work to be done with the animal models before we reach
the stage at which we can design appropriate experiments.

As gene therapy is perfected, and as more is learnt about gene
regulation in the transgenic mouse model, we may be tempted to
do transfer experiments using human fertilized ova. Here we
would be moving into a completely different area of research
because we would be manipulating genetic material which would
be passed on to subsequent generations. This would be dangerous
ground, and although we cannot imagine experiments of this type

being done in the foreseeable future it is a problem that we must keep in mind. Somatic cell gene therapy is only an extension of current medical practice; a transgenic man is another thing altogether.

Thus the major role for human embryos in human genetic research will be in developmental genetics. Until we know what questions to ask – and this information will gradually evolve from work with other species – it seems unlikely that this will be an active research field in the immediate future. However, it is one with considerable long-term potential, particularly for understanding the problems of congenital malformation, and therefore it should not be irrevocably closed.

References

Anderson, W.F. (1984) Prospects for human gene therapy. *Science* 226: 401–409.

Bishop, M.J. (1985) Viral oncogenes. *Cell* 42: 23–38

Cavanee, W.K., Dryja, T.P., Phillips, R.A., Benedict, W.F., Godbout, R., Gallie, B.L., Murphree, A.L., Strong, L.C., and White, R.L. (1983) Expression of recessive alleles by chromosomal mechanisms in retinoblastoma. *Nature* 305: 779–84

Collins, F.S. and Weismann, S.M. (1984) The molecular genetics of human hemoglobin. In W.E. Cohn and K. Moldave (eds) *Progress in Nucleic Acid Research and Molecular Biology* (31st edn). New York: Academic Press, pp. 315–462

Davies, K.E. (1985) Molecular genetics of the human X chromosome. *Journal of Medical Genetics* 22: 243–49

de la Chapelle, A. (1985) Mapping hereditary disorders. *Nature* 317: 472–73

Emery, A.E.H. (1984) *An Introduction to Recombinant DNA*. Chichester: Wiley

Gehring, W.J. (1985) The homeo box: a key to the understanding of development? *Cell* 40: 3–5

Gusella, J.F., Wexler, N.S., Conneally, P.M., Naylor, S.L., Anderson, M.A., Tanzi, R.E., Watkins, P.C., Ottina, K., Wallace, M.R., Sakayuchi, A.Y., Young, A.B., Shoulson, I., Bonilla, E., and Martin, J.B. (1983) A polymorphic DNA marker genetically linked to Huntington's disease. *Nature* 306: 234–38

Humphries, S.E., Kessling, A.M., Horsthemke, B., Seed, M., Jowett, N., Holm, M., Galton, D.J., Wynn, V., and Williamson, R. (1985) A common DNA polymorphism of the low-density lipoprotein (LDL) receptor gene and its use in diagnosis. *Lancet* 1: 1003–1005

Jeffreys, A.J., Wilson, V., and Thein, S.L. (1985) Hypervariable 'minisatellite' regions in human DNA. *Nature* 314: 67–73

Karanthanasis, S.K., McPherson, J., Zannis, V.I., and Breslow, J.L. (1983a) Linkage of human apolipoproteins A–I and C–III genes. *Nature* 304: 371–73

Karanthanasis, S.K., Norum, R.A., Zannis, V.I., and Breslow, J.L. (1983b) An inherited polymorphism in the human apolipoprotein A–I gene locus related to the development of atherosclerosis. *Nature* 301: 718–20

Latt, S.A., Kurnit, D.M., Bruns, G.P., Schreck, R.R., Morton, C.C., Kunkel, L.M., Lalande, M., Aldridge, J., Neve, R., Tantravahi, U. *et al.* (1984) Molecular genetic approaches to human diseases involving mental retardation. *American Journal of Mental Deficiency* 88: 561–71

Marx, J.L. (1985a) The cytochrome P450's and their genes. *Science* 228: 975–76

Marx, J.L. (1985b) Making mutant mice by gene transfer. *Science* 228: 1516–517

Orkin, S.H., Antonarakis, S.E., and Kazazian, H.H. (1983) Polymorphism and molecular pathology of the human beta-globin gene. In E.B. Brown (ed.) *Progress in Hematology* (13th edn). New York: Grune & Stratton, pp. 49–73

Palmiter, R.D. and Brinster, R.L. (1985) Transgenic mice. *Cell* 41: 343–45

Reeders, S.T., Breuning, M.H., Davies, K.E., Nicholls, R.D., Jarman, A.P., Higgs, D.R., Pearson, P.L., and Weatherall, D.J. (1985) A highly polymorphic DNA marker linked to adult polycystic kidney disease on chromosome 16. *Nature* 317: 542–44

Rees, A., Shoulders, C.G., Stocks, J., Galton, D.J., and Baralle, F.E. (1983) DNA polymorphism adjacent to human apoprotein A–I gene: relation to hypertriglyceridaemia. *Lancet* 1: 444–46

Smithies, O., Gregg, R.G., Boggs, S.S., Koralewski, M.A., and Kucherlapati, R.S. (1985) Insertion of DNA sequences into the human chromosomal β-globin locus by homologous recombination. *Nature* 317: 230–34

Sudhof, T.C., Goldstein, J.L., Brown, M.S., and Russell, D.W. (1985) The LDL receptor gene: a mosaic of exons shared with different proteins. *Science* 228: 815–22

Sutcliffe, J.C., Milner, R.J., Gottesfeld, J.M., and Reynolds, W. (1984) Control of neuronal gene expression. *Science* 225: 1308–315

Weatherall, D.J. (1985) *The New Genetics and Clinical Practice* (2nd edn). Oxford: Oxford University Press

Weatherall, D.J. and Wainscoat, J.S. (1985) The molecular pathology of thalassaemia. In A.V. Hoffbrand (ed.) *Recent Advances in Haematology* (4th edn). Edinburgh: Churchill Livingstone, pp. 63–108
Weatherall, D.J., Old, J.M., Thein, S.L., Wainscoat, J.S., and Clegg, J.B. (1985) Prenatal diagnosis of the common haemoglobin disorders. *Journal of Medical Genetics* 22: 422–30
Williams, D.A., Lemischka, I.R., Nathan, D.G., and Mulligan, R.C. (1984) Introduction of new genetic material into pluripotent haematopoietic stem cells of the mouse. *Nature* 310: 476–80

Discussion

Williamson: The amount of DNA needed for fairly reliable analysis is now down to 100 nanograms, or the amount in about one hundred thousand cells. A single chorionic villus contains about ten million cells, whereas the embryos Bob Edwards showed us contained eight cells. We are still only half-way to gene analysis at very early stages.

Weatherall: It is important to put this in context and to remember that chorionic villus sampling is not a traumatic procedure for pregnant women. But we don't yet know its long-term effects on the foetus.

Modell: It is important to point out why you have emphasized the DNA technology. Take thalassaemia (or sickle cell disease) as an example. Until the DNA technology was fully developed we couldn't test for this disease until the eighteenth week of pregnancy, when foetal blood samples can be taken safely. Then, if an affected foetus was diagnosed, the women had to choose whether or not to have the pregnancy terminated at about twenty weeks of pregnancy. Most couples were so afraid of having an affected child that they chose an abortion, which at that stage is a very stressful procedure, with a lot of psychological problems for the parents. The medical staff who see people through that kind of procedure cannot escape from the moral and emotional implications of such procedures. Though twenty-five per cent of the pregnant women at risk of having thalassaemic infants who came to us eventually had late abortions for thalassaemia, a surprisingly large number became pregnant again very soon. Two unfortunate women each had five antenatal diagnoses, and terminated four pregnancies at twenty weeks because of a positive diagnosis. These diseases can place a terrible burden on some people.

The introduction of DNA technology meant that if we could get *any* material at *any* stage after fertilization, and still preserve the embryo, we could make a diagnosis. Now the new DNA technology has been combined with the new obstetric technique of chorionic villus sampling at eight weeks of pregnancy, to provide much earlier antenatal diagnosis, and has proved extremely acceptable to our patients. When they heard that the new method was being developed some even decided not to get pregnant until we had perfected it. In collaboration with David Weatherall's group we now do 80 per cent of our diagnoses in the first trimester of pregnancy, and the transformation in what it means to the families to be able to have a genetic diagnosis at eight weeks instead of eighteen weeks is amazing.

Weatherall: Would there be any great advantage in being able to make a diagnosis even nearer the time of conception?

Modell: The United Kingdom Thalassaemia Society submitted their views on that to the Warnock Committee (Committee of Inquiry into Human Fertilisation and Embryology, 1982–1984). They said that their ideal would be to be able to start a pregnancy, knowing from the time of implantation that the foetus would be healthy. From the contrast between people's feelings about mid-trimester diagnosis and their feelings about first-trimester diagnosis, I now agree that for people at high genetic risk it would be a great benefit if the diagnosis could be made much earlier in pregnancy.

The World Health Organisation has been keeping an eye on the safety of first-trimester chorionic villus sampling by means of an international register. Over 8000 pregnancies have now undergone the procedure in 79 centres around the world. The average rate of foetal loss is about 4 per cent overall, and 2 per cent in those centres with most experience. It is still difficult to evaluate the meaning of these figures because we don't really know what the spontaneous abortion rate would be in a control group that had the same kind of ultrasound evaluation at the same stage in pregnancy, but no obstetric intervention. However, it seems possible that in good hands the technique has little more risk than that of amniocentesis.

Weatherall: We know that it works at the laboratory end in this country. We have had one technical mistake out of 115. We are now trying to set this technique up in large rural populations in the developing countries. The problems there are not technical but pastoral and organizational.

Edwards: We have tried one or two probes for typing pre-implantation embryos. The bkm probe from snake, made by Jones in Edinburgh, did bind to the mouse Y chromosome in tissue cells and the embryo. I believe this was tested on human cells but it did not attach to the Y chromosome *in situ*. We have also worked with Dr McGee in Oxford on another probe.

Why might such sequences be present in some species and not in others? What is the likelihood that such sequences could be used for hybridization *in situ*?

Weatherall: I would find it very difficult to envisage getting to the stage where one could diagnose single-gene disorders by *in situ* hybridization, certainly in the near future.

Williamson: Bkm is a snake sequence that can be used for DNA sexing. It is not a bad experiment if you are interested in snake sexing, but there are better human gene probes available. I shall be talking about DNA diagnosis at early stages later on [see Chapter 7].

Weatherall: One approach is to scale down the diagnostic techniques I have described and to develop techniques for the rapid culture of embryonic cells. It is now possible to synthesize short gene probes (oligonucleotides) that can identify single-base changes. A combination of these approaches might make it possible to identify single-gene disorders in cells from an early conceptus.

Williamson: You can analyse gene activity by hybridization to messenger RNA only if the gene is expressed at a fairly high level, which is not known at present for early embryos.

Edwards: I am not happy about the answer. If there was a Y probe, we could identify the presence of the Y sequence in an embryo. In sex-linked disorders there would be no need to find the haemophiliac gene, merely the Y chromosome.

Williamson: The families with sex-linked disorders are asking for the opportunity to have normal boys. For haemophilia we already have the ability to offer accurate antenatal diagnosis of whether the male foetus is affected or unaffected. When you only have a gene probe for foetal sexing, the families have to decide whether the pregnancy should be terminated even though the male foetus has a 50 per cent chance of being unaffected. This is what is less acceptable about offering only foetal sexing for X-linked diseases.

Edwards: There is a choice here: either abort all the afflicted and non-afflicted males or try restricting offspring to females, using blastocyst sexing. The all-female pregnancies in couples with sex-linked disorders would not result in an afflicted foetus. The alternative is to do chorionic villus sampling and abort the afflicted males. There is an ethical balance here, between the limitations to typing blasto-cysts versus the need to abort foetuses much later in gestation.

If we had a DNA probe for the long repeating sequences on chromosome 21, we might be able to type early embryos for their content of this chromosome. We would look for the presence of two chromosome 21s in the interphase nuclei of the early embryo without having to use karyotyping. If this approach proved feasible, we could get some idea of the incidence of trisomy in embryos by identifying three chromosome 21s. Otherwise, so many embryos are wasted because we karyotype them because they have no mitoses.

McLaren: David Weatherall asked what the benefit would be if these diagnoses could be made before implantation, on *in vitro* material. Infertile couples who are at high risk from some genetic disease or chromosomal disorder would certainly benefit. We are not necessarily envisaging people having IVF in order to be diagnosed but it must be a great anguish for an infertile couple of this kind to finally get pregnant and then to have the pregnancy terminated because the baby is affected.

Maddox: One way of dealing with the technology would then be to split the embryo at some point and grow half in the laboratory and the other half in the uterus.

McLaren: Bob Williamson may be talking about the technique of embryonic biopsy.

SEVEN

Research needs and the reduction of severe congenital disease

R. Williamson

Until recently, variation and pathology due to genetic causes, either alone or with environmental interaction, could only be studied in humans by classical inheritance analysis of family pedigrees, or by using animal models. Because of the power of recombinant DNA techniques, it is now possible to study human inheritance and development by examining gene organization and expression in single cells or organisms. Since genetic disease either directly or as a paradigm accounts for a high proportion of serious handicap in children and young adults, such studies may represent the only way to understand, and to prevent, many abnormalities. The study of early embryos may also be necessary if we are to understand the normal development of the foetus during pregnancy, and the development of the growing nervous system and the heart. While it is up to society as a whole to assess whether this information is to be obtained, there is no doubt that it would be of great and immediate clinical benefit if it were available.

It is difficult to overstate the revolution in medical research which has accompanied the general development of human molecular biology, in particular the isolation and analysis of genes by recombinant DNA techniques (Weatherall 1985). The first human genes were cloned a mere eight years ago (Little *et al.* 1978; Wilson *et al.* 1978) and over 300 coding genes and several thousand random DNA markers are now available (8th International Human Gene Mapping Workshop, Helsinki 1985). This has not only resulted in a vast increase in our knowledge of common inherited diseases but has also had two practical consequences – improvements in prevention and treatment of single-gene defects, and new approaches to polygenic conditions such as coronary heart disease which are common in middle life.

These achievements and possibilities have been commented on at length (Williamson 1985a, b; Weatherall 1985). In this chapter I wish instead to present my view of some of the information which might be obtained in the medium term (say, the next five to ten years) by research on embryos, and investigate the clinical consequences of this information and whether there are alternative ways of acquiring it.

I do this with some hesitation, since my own research group has not used normal human embryos and believes that many experiments can be done using foetal tissues obtained at termination of pregnancy, or using triploid embryos which are unsuitable for transfer (see p. 110). However, it is perhaps valuable to note the areas of research where such work may later become necessary if we are to reduce the incidence of handicap and inherited disease.

Congenital malformations and dysmorphologies

Connor and Ferguson-Smith, in their recently published textbook (1984), have estimated that about 3 per cent of newborn babies have a major deformity (dysmorphology), ranging from the relatively inconsequential (such as the extra fingers found in post-axial polydactyly, which are easily removed) to defects of the walls of the heart (septal defects) or to cleft palate, spina bifida, and mental retardation with associated physical signs. Such conditions almost invariably have a similar pattern of incidence – nearly all cases are sporadic but the frequency with which the defects occur is higher in first-degree relatives of those affected, and occasional families are found in which the condition is passed on in a simple Mendelian fashion.

The simplest explanation for this epidemiological pattern is that in such conditions there is interaction between more than one gene, and in some cases with environmental components as well. There is a comparable model about which we know more: heart disease in non-smokers below fifty-five years of age. Many cases are sporadic although the condition is almost entirely determined by the inheritance of about a dozen 'candidate genes' which code for the proteins, receptors, and enzymes controlling cholesterol metabolism and transport.

We use the term 'candidate gene' to refer to any gene where there is a biochemical or biological or genetic reason to suppose that the sequence causes or contributes to an inherited phenotype. The advantage of this approach is that it allows definitive experiments to be done using such genes to track risks in families.

Dysmorphologies are more complex than heart disease. From studies of twins we know that conditions do not always occur in both of a pair of identical twins. This demonstrates that environmental as well as genetic factors must be involved. Also, we understand little of what kinds of genes regulate form, so we find it difficult to comprehend what type of DNA mutation can cause a congenital malformation. By analogy with diseases that are truly polygenic, the genetic analysis of dysmorphology can be regarded as the search for candidate genes such as those in which a mutation will cause, say, a 'hole in the heart' to develop.

Some of the genes that modulate human development will be the analogues of homoeotic genes in *Drosophila*. These have recently been identified because mutations cause dysmorphologies, often in fundamental segmentation – that is, arms, legs, wings, and genitalia appear in inappropriate numbers or places because of errors during embryonic development. Similar sequences, which also code for proteins expressed during early development, occur in mammals, including humans. One might predict that at least some human dysmorphologies, such as those where limbs are altered or absent, are due to mutations in these genes. Other inherited or multifactorial conditions, such as polydactyly, might involve mutations in or close to sequences that determine the activity of cell-specific growth factors and receptors which control cell proliferation and orientation during embryogenesis. These are the sorts of candidate genes which clinical scientists wish to study during embryonic development.

Since it is possible to study such genes in animals, whether mice or fruit flies, why bother to study either human families or human embryos? Consider polydactyly as a model. There are families in which an extra finger occurs, inherited as a Mendelian dominant. Because a total human gene map is now almost available (White 1985), it should soon be possible to determine by linkage which chromosomal region is co-segregating with polydactyly and then, by walking along the chromosome, find the actual gene that is mutated.

Once this gene has been found it will be possible to determine its normal function – when it is expressed in embryonic development, which cells it regulates, and when and how it is turned off to prevent us having too many fingers. It will also be possible to compare this site of action with the effects of other agents, such as viruses and teratogens, which also cause polydactyly. In this way we should be able to stop these substances in the environment coming into contact with pregnant women at the relevant times during embryogenesis.

Cleft palate and other mid-line defects provide a further good example of the way in which an extremely rare family showing Mendelian inheritance may help in the future to increase our understanding of genetic and environmental causes of this class of morphological disability. There are families in which cleft palate segregates as a sex-linked recessive – only males who are affected (50 per cent of the males in the family) develop secondary cleft palate, while female carriers develop a minor condition known as ankyloglossia in which they are 'tongue-tied' at birth. Sex-linked cleft palate is rare, as evidenced by the fact that it is almost as common amongst girls as boys. However, the X-chromosome has been completely mapped with linked markers, over 150 in all, which will allow the defect in this particular family to be located.

If the family wish, they can have antenatal diagnosis of affected pregnancies using these gene probes as linked markers. However, the real value will be our ability to determine the mechanism of action of the gene defect, throwing light on the much more common sporadic cases of cleft palate where genetic and environmental causes interact.

It should perhaps be noted here that organogenesis – whether we are studying limb formation as in polydactyly, the heart in septum defects, or the nervous system – for the most part occurs at between fourteen and twenty-eight days of embryonic development. It is this area of research, which is central to the understanding of congenital malformation, which in my view would be most inhibited were a strict fourteen-day rule to be implemented.

The uniqueness of human development

How unique is human development? Obviously, all mammals share features of embryogenesis. However, it is also obvious that some aspects of gene expression and determination are not common to all species. This is perhaps most apparent when we consider the brain and nervous system. Since so much handicap is determined developmentally in the nervous system (for instance, neuronal sensory deafness is produced by defects in migration of cells of the neural crest), it is hard to see how handicap of this kind can be studied without using human material, at least in small amounts. One reason why human material will be required is that most experimental laboratory animals are inbred populations, while humans are decidedly outbred.

Consider one of the most important clinical phenotypes – trisomy 21 or Down's syndrome – which is the most common defined cause of mental retardation in the United Kingdom. There are several questions which can be asked. The first is, why do the chromosome pairs fail to separate properly (non-disjunction) in the first place? This can be studied using cloned gene probes for chromosome 21, as we showed two years ago (Davies *et al.* 1984). I would venture to guess, although there is little evidence one way or the other at this time, that non-disjunction is under genetic control and that some families are particularly prone to this anomaly. Normally, non-disjunction is not detected because it leads to a non-viable foetus, unless chromosome 21 is affected.

An equally important question relates to the nature of the changes that occur during embryogenesis and result in the physical signs of Down's syndrome. Why does an extra copy of chromosome 21 give the characteristic facial features of the Down's child, the fingerprints, the heart malformations, and the early brain changes at the age of thirty that are so reminiscent of

Alzheimer's disease? Are each of these the result of the activity of a single extra gene or of several genes working together? One way to study this crucial set of questions is to examine gene expression and development of trisomic embryonic material *in vitro*.

Fortunately, this kind of study may be possible ethically. When ova are fertilized *in vitro*, it often happens that two sperm enter a single egg, giving a triploid embryo. Such an embryo is non-viable, and no one would reimplant it. However, it develops more or less normally in culture up to the late blastocyst stage, and it seems that many questions about gene activity can be answered with such material.

Gene expression in early human embryos

It is thought that there are about 100000 coding genes in the human genome, although only a tenth of this number are expressed in most tissues. A higher proportion are expressed in the early mammalian embryo. Surprisingly, we understand little about the roles of most of these genes. The fact that they are found as messenger RNA transcripts implies that they code for proteins.

Some aspects of gene expression are of great importance clinically. For instance, we understand little of the timing or nature of expression of cell surface antigens during early foetal life. One cause of infertility is immunological rejection of the foetus by the mother but the precise foetal determinants involved have not been defined. Such studies require gene transcripts from embryos at different developmental stages, although of course these can be from terminations of pregnancy rather than from embryos obtained by *in vitro* fertilization (IVF). Embryonic gene expression and its control are of course also related to the problem of cancer, in which cells often revert to a foetal protein pattern. The identification of proteins expressed during early foetal development is also seen as one of the most promising approaches to the development of vaccines which control fertility in man (Ada, Basten, and Jones 1985).

We have recently become interested in the timing of gene expression in early embryos. The expression of some foetal hormones has previously been studied at the protein level, and can now be investigated by looking directly at gene transcripts as

well (Vasseur, Condamine, and Duprey 1985; Craig and Williamson 1986). In this way we may gain understanding of the reasons
underlying recurrent abortion in some women and placental
insufficiency in others.

Mental handicap and single-gene defects

The prevention and treatment of mental handicap is a priority for
the National Health Service in the UK and is also under intensive
investigation in many other countries. There are several specific
causes of mental handicap, some of which (such as birth trauma)
are clearly preventable and not genetic. However, the majority of
cases are either genetic, or sporadic but with an increased
incidence in close family members.

I have already discussed the most common cause of mental
retardation, Down's syndrome. Here I shall focus on simple and
complex conditions involving one or a small number of gene
alterations. Mental retardation sometimes occurs as a consequence of a metabolic defect; the paradigm is phenylketonuria,
an autosomal recessive disease in which the amino acid phenyl-
alanine cannot be converted to tyrosine. We know how to
prevent this condition by altering the diet of affected infants, but
we still have few ideas on how the mental retardation is caused,
nor do we know if the residual learning disabilities (within the
normal range) faced by treated children with phenylketonuria are
a result of developmental problems during foetal life. This is a key
question in the management of patients since, if it arises during
development, phenylketonuria may be best treated before birth
rather than after.

There are several other examples. Huntington's disease is
caused by a defect in a single gene and it manifests itself with a set
of bizarre psychiatric and motor symptoms at about the age of
forty-five years. Alzheimer's disease has a strong familial ten-
dency, as do psychotic diseases such as schizophrenia. For
conditions such as this, the general objective of clinicians is *not* to
perform antenatal diagnosis or (even less) to contemplate gene
therapy, but to use knowledge of the molecular basis of the
disease to predict those who are at risk and devise new methods
for prevention and treatment.

Gene analysis and gene therapy

Until recently, antenatal diagnosis of inherited biochemical disease, such as haemophilia or mucopolysaccharidoses, or of chromosomal abnormalities such as Down's syndrome, had to take place at about nineteen weeks of pregnancy. If the diagnosis predicted an affected foetus, the pregnancy could be terminated at the parent's request at about twenty weeks, a very upsetting event for the mother, for both medical and social reasons. The time of diagnosis has now been moved back to nine weeks of pregnancy for many disorders by the use of chorion villus sampling (Williamson *et al.* 1981).

Although this is a marked and much appreciated advance, there are still many women, particularly from the group who object to abortion, who would prefer antenatal diagnosis even earlier in pregnancy. There is a real demand for diagnosis of affected foetuses [early embryos] during the preimplantation stages of pregnancy, particularly after IVF. These techniques of gene analysis can be pioneered with animal models but, if they are to be applied, they must ultimately be proven with human material.

In addition to those couples who might choose IVF so that they can have antenatal diagnosis before implantation and so avoid the possibility of termination at later stages of pregnancy, there are also couples who now request IVF for infertility and are at risk of inherited disease. For instance, one person in twenty is a carrier of the gene defect causing cystic fibrosis. There is also the possibility of Down's syndrome in IVF children; the mothers are often in the at-risk older group, and several such children have been conceived already.

What we would like to do is ensure that any fertilized ovum reimplanted in a mother is normal chromosomally and genetically, as nearly as this can be determined. At present we cannot do this because we do not know how to isolate the small numbers of foetal cells needed for such analyses. Therefore, it is important, for the safety and health of the reimplanted embryo, to devise techniques for the tissue culture of disaggregated embryonic cells and single cells from the morula and blastocyst stages, and for activating specific genes in embryonic cells so that we can determine whether they function normally.

There is also a demand from families for gene surgery (what I have called somatic gene therapy: Williamson 1981) to correct organ systems that have gone wrong for genetic reasons. The most obvious examples are from among the haemoglobinopathies, where red blood cell precursors in the marrow cannot make appropriate amounts of haemoglobin. This might be corrected by the insertion of a normal globin gene into marrow stem cells, which would then function well enough to correct the severe anaemia (Smithies *et al.* 1985). Foetal life is the obvious time to attempt such correction, as there ought to be fewer immunological problems. Once again experiments with both animal models and human material will be necessary before such techniques can be tried on those suffering from these conditions.

Somatic gene therapy, where a gene is placed in cells of a relevant tissue but not in gametes, should not be confused with genetic therapy. It is not possible at present to insert genes into early embryos in such a way as to alter the inheritance (as opposed to the phenotype) of an individual, nor is it likely to become possible in the foreseeable future. Such gene manipulation would have to be far more sophisticated than is now possible, since it is probably necessary to excise precisely the non-functional gene as well as insert the normal one, perhaps on two chromosomes of a pair simultaneously. Leaving aside any questions of public policy, gene-level gene therapy is not an issue today, because no one is even close to making it work for diseases such as thalassaemia or the haemophilias.

Conclusion

The entire concept of 'inherited disease' is changing as we realize that many common conditions are due to an interaction between *specific* gene determinants and agents in the general environment. Conditions affecting morphology and the development of the nervous system occur, for the most part, during embryogenesis. If the incidence of these conditions is to be reduced, we must learn more about gene structure, expression, and interaction during foetal life. While many of these findings can be made using animal models or material obtained from terminations of pregnancy, some could be best verified using foetal material obtained from IVF. Often triploid (pathological) material will be suitable but occasionally, particularly if a finding is to be used as a starting point for clinical treatment, it may be necessary to use normal material at early stages of pregnancy.

There seems no scientific reason to draw an absolute line to stop studies of embryonic material at fourteen days, since each case could be judged on its merits. To insist on ethical scrutiny is essential, but to place laws around scientific experimentation could make it more difficult to use the techniques of molecular genetics to study and reduce human handicap and illness.

References

Ada, G.L., Basten, A., and Jones, W.R. (1985) Prospects for developing vaccines to control fertility. *Nature* 317: 288–89

Craig, F. and Williamson, R. (1986) Gene expression in human chorionic villi. *Human Reproduction* 1: in press

Connor, J.M. and Ferguson-Smith, M.A. (1984) *Essential Medical Genetics.* Oxford: Blackwell Scientific Publications

Davies, K.E., Harper, K., Bonthron, D., Krumlauf, R., Polkey, A., Pembrey, M.E., and Williamson, R. (1984) Use of a chromosome 21 cloned DNA probe for the analysis of non-disjunction in Down syndrome. *Human Genetics* 66: 54–6

8th International Human Gene Mapping Workshop, Helsinki (1985) *Cytogenetics and Cell Genetics*, vol. 40

Little, P.F.R., Curtis, P., Coutelle, C.H., Van den Berg, J., Dalgleish, R., Malcolm, S., Courtney, M., Westaway, D., and Williamson, R. (1978) Isolation and partial sequence of recombinant plasmids containing human α-, β- and γ-globin cDNA fragments. *Nature* 273: 640–43

Smithies, O., Gregg, R.G., Boggs, S.S., Koralewski, M.A., and Kucherlapati, R.S. (1985) Insertion of DNA sequences into the human chromosomal β-globin locus by homologous recombination. *Nature* 317: 230–34

Vasseur, M., Condamine, H., and Duprey, P. (1985) RNAs containing B2 repeated sequences are transcribed in the early stages of mouse embryogenesis. *EMBO (European Molecular Biology Organization) Journal* 4: 1749–753

Weatherall, D.J. (1985) *The New Genetics and Clinical Practice* (2nd edn). Oxford: Oxford University Press

White, R. (1985) DNA sequence polymorphisms revitalize linkage approaches in human genetics. *Trends in Genetics* 1: 177–81

Williamson, R. (1981) Gene therapy. *Nature* 298: 416–18

Williamson, R. (1985a) Cloned genes and their use in the analysis of inherited disease. *Biochemical Society Transactions* 13: 808–11

Williamson, R. (1985b) Towards a total human gene map: the Woodhull Lecture. *Proceedings of the Royal Institution of Great Britain* 57: 45–55

Williamson, R., Eskdale, J., Coleman, D.V., Niazi, M., Loeffler, F.E., and Modell, B.M. (1981) Direct gene analysis of chorionic villi: a possible technique for first-trimester antenatal diagnosis of haemoglobinopathies. *Lancet* 2: 1125–127

Wilson, J.T., Wilson, L.B., deRiel, J.K., Villa-Komaroff, L., Efstratiadis, A., Forget, B.G., and Weissman, S.M. (1978) Insertion of synthetic copies of human globin genes into bacterial plasmids. *Nucleic Acids Research* 5: 563–81

Discussion

Casey: How imminent are experiments on normal human material obtained after IVF in the twelve to twenty-four-day period you have been speaking about? I understand that embryos have not yet been kept alive to that developmental stage.

Williamson: Probably no one has tried because of doubts about its acceptability to the community and to our colleagues, as well as for technical reasons. I have never done an experiment on a normal human embryo.

Dunstan: Now that we have heard Bob Williamson talk about preventive work at the pre-embryo stage as a preferred alternative to late abortion would you consider the wisdom and the prudence of using (as you have) the word 'abortion' for pre-embryonic selection, Professor Edwards? Philologically abortion means the ejection of an immature foetus from the uterus. If the foetus is not there, there is a philological reason for avoiding the word. Emotionally and morally as well as logically its use invites a wrong response to what you are doing.

Edwards: I fully agree. It is important to clarify the nomenclature. The same thing arose with the term 'spare embryo', and we were advised not to use that either. We wished to draw attention to the abnormality of these embryos, and a better term would be 'spontaneous abortion *in vitro'*. A spontaneous abortion is very different from an induced abortion.

Dunstan: But the pre-embryos you use have never gone into the uterus: they cannot logically, therefore, be 'aborted'.

Edwards: I take that point.

The bkm probe mentioned earlier could be used for sexing in mouse embryos and *Drosophila*, not just snakes. There are nucleotide sequences that are common to all these species and I think its use should be encouraged. Howard Jacobs told us about getting twenty embryos from some patients by modern techniques. If these were fertilized, it might be possible to identify ten embryos with and ten without the risk of sex-linked disorders, by means of sexing. These techniques are being developed very quickly and we should not close our eyes to them.

Braude: It is certainly dangerous to believe that if we don't have the technology now it is not going to be available very soon. Five years ago we were told it was impossible to look at messenger RNA or embryonic proteins because we would have to use large numbers of embryos. Now we can use single embryos or indeed single cells. One can envisage doing this kind of work on a biopsy of an embryo, for example, rather than on a whole embryo. One might remove one of the embryonic cells, grow it and work on the cell line, perhaps freezing the other three cells from the pre-embryo. How would that fall within the moral understanding of what a pre-embryo is? If we can grow that single cell, or two cells out of four, would we have to give them some moral status? How much of the pre-embryo could be taken for this kind of work without its becoming morally offensive?

Dunstan: The organism is then at such a fluid stage that it has not yet the individuality necessary to be counted a person in a legal sense, or even the substantial basis for a legal person. You are still dealing with some pre-identifiably human stage of cellular development. At what point in the development of such an organism a biopsy becomes an interruption is a question which only the scientists can answer.

Braude: Is this experimental research or diagnosis?

Dunstan: I don't want to label this now but it seems to me that if you are able to take a cell from the organism without destroying the organism, that organism is not yet fixed – it is not yet an individual.

Maddox: This is a dangerous path for scientists to follow. Anne McLaren pointed out that we go through a continuous cycle, and your definition would put a term to what Anne would call the onset of commitment at about four days, Professor Dunstan. If one accepts that the cycle is continuous, one has no alternative but to accept the same interdictions on embryos as one does on adults. If, on the other hand, one recognizes that the interdiction on killing adults derives from all kinds of social considerations, such as that it would be very dangerous to live in a society in which it is permissible, the interdiction on what is done with embryos is of quite a different order. Unless one makes that distinction one is tied up with these constant problems that Warnock got into with fourteen days and so on.

McLaren: The technique of embryonic biopsy is important if one wants to diagnose genetic defects in the preimplantation period. Taking one cell from a four-cell stage or an eight-cell stage, or taking a small group of cells from a blastocyst, provided that it doesn't prejudice the future development of the rest of the pre-embryo or conceptus, is very much like taking a tissue sample from an adult for diagnostic purposes, which is done all the time. However, at present we don't know at what stages one can take an embryonic biopsy and how many cells one can remove without prejudicing further development. If the method is to be pursued, that will have to be found out by the sort of experiment that Peter Braude was telling us about earlier.

Secondly, we don't know the best methods for growing the few cells that have been removed in order to get enough DNA to make the diagnoses that Bob Williamson was telling us about. Bob mentioned the possibility of switching on the genes so that the messenger RNA can be identified, but it may also be possible to make the diagnosis directly on the DNA to see whether the normal or the abnormal gene is there. Some of that work is done on animals now but if the method is to be used clinically the later stages will have to be done on human material.

Johnson:　I agree, but if legislation is going to be drawn up to regulate this kind of work, it must make clear what constitutes a biopsy. For example, it is possible to take one or two cells from a four-cell pre-embryo as a biopsy, but the single cell or the pair of cells can also give rise to a complete embryo subsequently. This is one way in which identical twins arise. So which is the biopsy and which is the pre-embryo? Should one pre-embryo be regarded as one, two, or more potential embryos? If only one, then biopsies should be permitted, since development of the remaining cells will not be prejudiced. If more than one, then biopsies clearly cannot be allowed.

Iglesias:　If the being that is generated at conception is an organic whole, and if the cells taken for biopsy at very early stages can give rise to a human being, a new whole, this fragmentation is another form of generation. I would object to that because the new being is not given the chance to live, and the fragmentation may not be beneficial for the first generated embryo. Later on, if there is no damage to the embryo, I do not think there would be any objection to biopsy if it is done for the benefit of the individual being.

Braude:　So you would only be prepared to take a piece of the early embryo if it was after the stage at which it had differentiated and that piece could no longer become another being?

Iglesias:　Yes. And if there were no damage.

Baird:　But the remaining bit would not benefit because the only reason for doing a biopsy, if the embryo was abnormal, would be to terminate its life.

Iglesias:　Then I wouldn't take it.

Edwards:　Bob Williamson made an eloquent plea for going beyond fourteen days because we cannot draw an arbitrary line. I happen to share that opinion but this is a major decision to make. We have to decide who would give consent and how we get that consent. Would you be prepared to grow an embryo beyond day fourteen if you thought the purpose was sufficiently important, Professor Williamson?

Williamson: I hope I did not make an eloquent plea for going beyond fourteen days; the point I was trying to make is that it is very difficult to draw an arbitrary line from the biological or clinical point of view. Personally, I am not an absolutist when it comes to ethics. I regard all human material as of value, and I would not do any experiments that I regard as unnecessary or wasteful either before or after fourteen days. All experiments should be judged both by import and intent.

If there is an important question which can only be answered using later material, and if this would result in major benefits to the patients and families with whom I work, I would certainly consider doing such work, particularly with material that would otherwise be discarded. There are experiments on primates that I regard as being far less ethical than some of the experiments that we are discussing. I do not agree with an absolutist ethical line, whether in terms of time or in terms of species. There are genuine ethical considerations but they should be looked at case by case.

Edwards: We might wish to do some work after day fourteen on the differentiation of tissues. Some could be important clinically. Should we do such work? It seems always as if the ethics follows the technology. It is always a scientist or a doctor who has to make these decisions.

Clothier: Ethics in a sense is your particular private law. Then there is a substantive law which follows on even further behind when public opinion crystallizes in favour of some sort of rule. Engraving laws in tablets of stone without any consultation is not possible in a civilized society. The trouble is that the law has fallen too far behind and that is causing anxiety.

Edwards: There have been examples where an organization took on collective responsibility for sensitive matters of this kind.

Williamson: The Genetic Manipulation Advisory Group (GMAG) did so in its early days.

Bowker: Religions that have clear understandings of when human life begins would paradoxically want to resist setting any sort of arbitrary date to this kind of work. They would take the view that if it is human material you don't treat it lightly; but you *may* actually treat it, in some circumstances.

Baird: None of us would suggest using a newborn baby for experimental purposes but experiments are done with newborn babies. They have to be done or infant mortality would still be 300 per thousand. It depends on how you define an experiment. It is probably justified to take a smear from a baby or a small sample of its blood if the yield from the observations is sufficiently good in relation to the risk the baby undergoes. The baby is not in a position to give informed consent at that stage. Society at present tolerates these experiments on babies, who in this respect do not differ qualitatively from the human embryo.

Clothier: The word 'experiment' has unfortunate connotations. These are really trials with an uncertain outcome, aren't they?

Iglesias: The difference is that in morally acceptable experiments you know you will not deliberately harm or destroy the baby.

Baird: This kind of experiment is done with the knowledge that there might under some circumstances be a very small risk to the baby. It is a quantitative difference.

Maddox: In the Medical Research Council's trials on spina bifida or neural tube defects the object was to discover whether vitamins, particularly folic acid, affected the development of these conditions. The trials were controversial because many people said that the question was already settled and it would be wrong to have a control group of women at risk of carrying damaged children. The experiment nevertheless went ahead. At some point somebody will probably be able to use living human embryos to discover whether folic acid has the predicted effects at about twenty or thirty days. Then the MRC would be taken off the hook it was on a couple of years ago.

McLaren: Bob Williamson mentioned the possibility of a normal gene being inserted instead of a defective gene in preimplantation stages. As he said, the technology for that is a long way ahead. In my view it would be a daft thing to do anyway. In every genetic or chromosomal defect that one knows about, a couple will produce normal conceptuses as well as defective ones. If you can diagnose which is which, it seems pointless to try to insert normal genes at this stage.

Modell: The impression I get is that everyone is supporting the Warnock Committee's main recommendation for an advisory committee to which individual experiments can be referred.

EIGHT

Human embryo research: the case for contraception

R.J. Aitken and D.W. Lincoln

Human *in vitro* fertilization (IVF) affords a hitherto unavailable step in the development of new approaches to contraception, falling between animal studies on the one hand and phase 1 clinical trials on the other. Studies using human gametes, and occasionally IVF, could provide important information on the mechanism of action, efficacy, and safety of new methods designed to render spermatozoa and oocytes incapable of achieving fertilization. Much of this information can be obtained using *in vitro* tests of sperm function, including the interspecies fertilization test, and through the use of oocytes, obtained from non-human species, that express immunological determinants similar to those of humans. As a final step, however, limited studies using human IVF would be desirable – although if a contraceptive method failed at this stage a human embryo would be produced. An answer to this dilemma might be provided by a definition of fertilization which takes into account the duration and complexity of the process. For most investigations, development could be arrested at the pronuclear stage, when the male and female pronuclei are still separate and the cell is functioning biochemically on the maternal genetic material (messenger RNA) derived during oocyte development.

The limiting resource in these and similar studies is the supply of oocytes. If women are allowed to donate oocytes for research, should these be used for studies designed to procure safer and more effective methods of contraception, or for studies related to infertility or congenital defects? The number of embryos wasted by the termination of unwanted pregnancies exceeds by five orders of magnitude the number produced by IVF for all purposes on a world scale.

The *in vitro* fertilization/embryo transfer (IVF/ET) procedure was originally devised as a treatment for infertility in women, particularly those in whom both Fallopian tubes were blocked. We have now come to realize that this technique has other applications, notably in the study, diagnosis, and treatment of genetic disorders, and in the development of new approaches to contraception. In the latter case, the ability to fertilize the human egg *in vitro*, study its growth in the following days, and determine its chromosomal make-up (karyotype) provides an intermediate step in contraceptive development between studies on animals and the use of human subjects.

IVF and the evaluation of contraceptive methods

The two most commonly used techniques for preventing conception are the contraceptive pill, which acts to prevent follicle growth and ovulation, and the condom, which provides a physical barrier that serves to contain spermatozoa. Several new approaches to contraception seek to change the hormonal environment in women in more subtle ways (e.g. with the progesterone-only mini-pill [Graham and Fraser 1982] and anti-progestagen [Healy and Fraser 1985]) or to render the spermatozoa functionally incompetent (e.g. with systemic agents such as gossypol or spermicides).

Much effort is now devoted to the development of gamete-specific toxins that might be taken orally to impair sperm production or render the spermatozoa functionally incapable of fertilizing an oocyte (Fong 1984). Likewise it might be possible, after further research, to convert spermicides from 'detergents' into agents capable of selectively impairing sperm function. In this context, a range of sperm function tests has been developed, based on the analysis of sperm number, morphology, and motility, as well as their ability to penetrate cervical mucus and salt-stored zonae pellucidae. The fertilizing potential of human spermatozoa can also be effectively assessed by examining their capacity to fuse with the vitelline membrane of zona-free hamster oocytes (Aitken *et al.* 1983). This test will have a pivotal role in screening chemical agents that might prevent fertilization (Yanagimachi, Yanagimachi, and Rogers 1976). The technique presents no ethical problems because the genetic disparity between the human and hamster genotypes means there is absolutely no possibility that human/hamster hybrids can be produced. In the past, when a potential chemical was found that acted as an effective contraceptive in animal studies and that passed toxicological tests, one would have sought to use the chemical in a limited clinical trial and trust that this did not lead to unwanted pregnancies or to abnormalities in the offspring. Is it not now logical to explore in a limited study the ability of any selected agents to block human IVF, and to determine, if the agents fail to work, the normality of the embryonic karyotype (Angell *et al.* 1983) that results? This experimental production of embryos, albeit as a consequence of failure, might be deemed unacceptable. However, this has to be balanced against the need for contraception and the risks of increasing early embryonic losses and, at worst, producing congenital defects.

Gamete-specific antigens and contraceptive vaccines

Contraceptive vaccines are now a realistic proposition, given the recent advances in recombinant DNA technology and peptide synthesis (Ada, Basten, and Jones 1985). Such vaccines would be an extremely welcome addition to our contraceptive armamentarium, particularly in developing countries where an infrastructure exists for the administration of vaccines against disease. They might even find acceptability amongst couples in developed countries seeking long-term contraception in the post-family years. Clearly such a vaccine would have to target a specific antigen which was present either transiently or in low amounts, or both, and which played a critical role during either fertilization or the early stages of embryonic development. The immunogenicity of the selected antigen would also be critical, as would its sensitivity to immunological attack. Ideally one would hope to identify a very immunogenic molecule, the biological function of which could be neutralized by low levels of antibody. In such a situation one would hope to achieve prolonged and efficient protection against conception, irrespective of differences between recipients in race, health, or nutritional status. In ideal circumstances the protective effect of the vaccine should also be reversible, either spontaneously (in which case protocols for monitoring antibody levels would have to be developed) or by artificial means.

The search for an antigen possessing these properties has focused on the male and female gametes (the spermatozoon or ovum) as well as on the early stages of development. Gamete-specific antigens probably constitute the most acceptable target, because a vaccine targeting these cells would have the effect of blocking conception.

As an example, take the development of a vaccine which targets the human spermatozoon. The contraceptive potential of anti-sperm antibodies is indicated by a wealth of clinical information indicating that the development of immunity against sperm antigens is a contributory factor in both male and female infertility (Aitken 1982) (Fig. 8.1). In the male, autoantibodies may be detected in the seminal plasma and in the peripheral circulation as the product of local and systemic immune reactions, respectively, but clearly it is the antibodies in the seminal plasma which are most relevant to fertility. These antibodies appear to be generated within the male reproductive tract, frequently in association with local infections or as a result of local trauma, the most common cause of which is vasectomy. These locally produced antibodies coat the spermatozoa and block their potential for fertilization either by inhibiting the progress of these cells through the female reproductive tract or by disrupting their capacity to fertilize the ovum. In a similar manner the presence of anti-sperm antibodies in infertile women is thought to block fertility by impeding the transport of spermatozoa to the site of fertilization as well as the act of fertilization itself. The inhibition of sperm transport is particularly apparent at the level of the cervix where the presence of immunoglobulin A (IgA) class anti-sperm antibodies, either in the mucus or on the sperm surface, impedes the progress of the spermatozoa through the channels between the mucin chains. In contrast the disruption of fertiliz-ation depends on the identity of the sperm surface antigens being targeted by such antibodies rather than the class to which the antibodies belong.

The surface of the human spermatozoon contains a vast array of antigenic components, only a fraction of which are critical to the process of fertilization. In order to develop a contraceptive

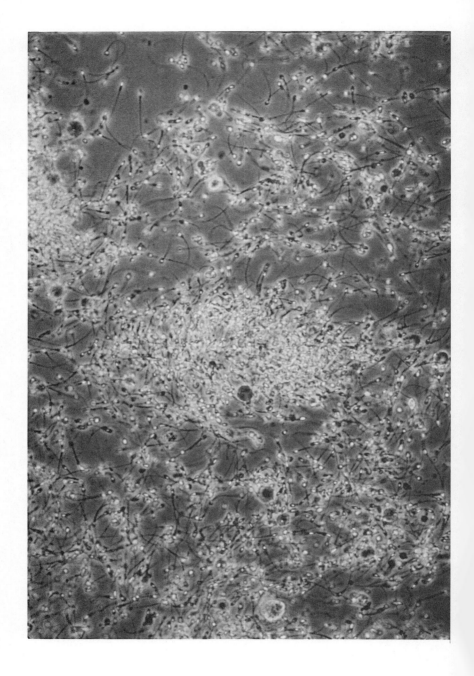

vaccine based on anti-sperm antibodies, we need to identify which of these surface components are involved in the major events of cell recognition associated with fertilization. There are two such events which might be blocked by anti-sperm antibodies for contraceptive purposes. The first of these is the binding of the spermatozoon to a clear acellular shell which surrounds the oocyte, the zona pellucida (Figs. 8.2 and 8.3). On its outermost surface the zona pellucida contains receptors-for-sperm which interact with complementary receptors on the surface of the spermatozoa. This interaction is extremely species-specific, which means that only the human zona pellucida can be used to assess the ability of any potential vaccine to block this stage of fertilization.

The ability of anti-zona antibodies to block the fertilization of ova *in vivo* and *in vitro* has been known for about ten years (Aitken, Richardson, and Hulme 1984). Such antibodies also achieve their effect by blocking the ability of the spermatozoa to recognize the sperm receptor sites on the surface of the zona pellucida. The anti-zona antibodies achieve this effect by inducing an immunoprecipitation layer to form at the zona surface; this layer then masks the receptors-for-sperm by steric hindrance (Fig. 8.3). As the antigens of which the zona pellucida is composed are known to be extremely specific, the induction of immunity against this material is unlikely to produce any side-effects that are due to cross-reactivity with other tissues. Furthermore, studies in animals such as the rat and marmoset monkey indicate that the induction of active immunity against the zona pellucida is compatible with the expression of long-term infertility free from obvious harmful side-effects. The development of a strategy for turning these promising studies in animals into a contraceptive vaccine has rested on the key observation that antibodies raised against the zona pellucida of the pig will both bind to the human zona and prevent the fertilization of human oocytes *in vitro*. Peptides isolated from the pig zona pellucida are therefore being used as the raw material for engineering a vaccine for human use.

Figure 8.1 clumping (autoagglutination) of spermatozoa in the ejaculate of a patient who has developed a state of autoimmunity against sperm antigens

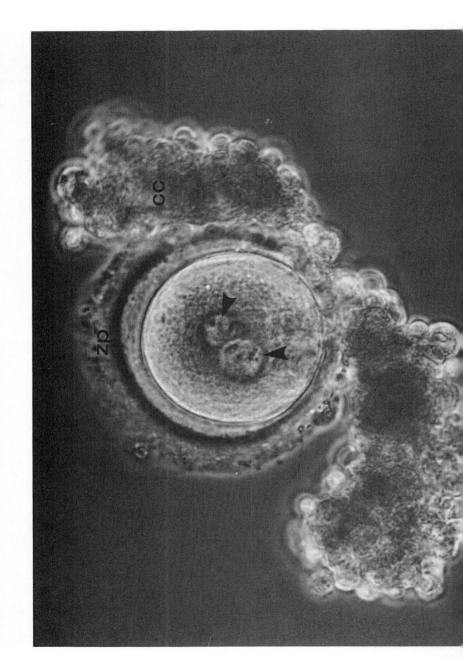

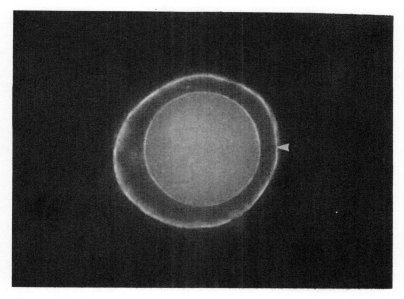

Figure 8.3   immunoprecipitation layer (arrowed) formed on the outer surface of the zona pellucida in the presence of anti-zona antibodies

Once again the species-specificity of sperm–zona interaction means that the final test of any anti-zona vaccine would be its ability to block fertilization *in vitro*.

The development of techniques for assessing this sperm–zona interaction need not pose an ethical problem since the zonae pellucidae surrounding non-viable oocytes can still interact normally with human spermatozoa (Yanagimachi *et al.* 1979) and such non-viable ova could be obtained from organ donors after death. Alternatively, viable ova could be recovered from donors at laparoscopy and then transferred to a specially designed culture medium with a high salt concentration. This medium

Figure 8.2   human embryo, pronucleate stage, showing the two pronuclei (arrowed), the zona pellucida (zp) and remnants of the cumulus cells (cc) which, before fertilization, completely encase the ovum

destroys the oocyte but preserves the structural integrity and biological properties of the zona pellucida. The availability of such material will be a critical factor in the development of contraceptive vaccines. It will be of value not only in testing the effectiveness of vaccines directed against the spermatozoon but also in the development of vaccines targeting the zona pellucida itself.

Once the human spermatozoon has penetrated the zona pellucida it must then recognize and fuse with the plasma membrane of the oocyte. This recognition event is also susceptible to interference by anti-sperm antibodies. Indeed, antibodies recovered from infertile men and women have a unique capacity to interfere with this stage of fertilization (Dor, Rudak, and Aitken 1981). The ability of antibodies to inhibit sperm–oocyte fusion need not, at least in the first instance, be assessed in human gametes. Instead, zona-free hamster oocytes can be used in an interspecies test of the fertilizing potential of human spermatozoa, as previously discussed (p. 123) (Fig. 8.4).

In the first instance, therefore, the development of contraceptive vaccines based on gamete-specific antigens need not present any major ethical problems since no human embryos would have been created in the process. Instead, salt-stored human zonae pellucidae and hamster oocytes could have been used to assess the influence of contraceptive antibodies on the key recognition events associated with fertilization. Valuable as such techniques are, they still constitute only a first step in the evaluation of a contraceptive vaccine. Before such an approach reaches the stage of a clinical trial, the ability of the vaccine to disrupt the fertilization of an intact human ovum *in vitro* should be ascertained, although failure in this test would still lead to the production of a human embryo.

Fertilization and the development of an embryo

An ethical dilemma therefore arises if new forms of contraception eventually have to be tested for their ability to block human *in vitro* fertilization. How could this be done without running the risk of creating a human embryo? The answer could rest on the development of a more precise definition of fertilization that takes

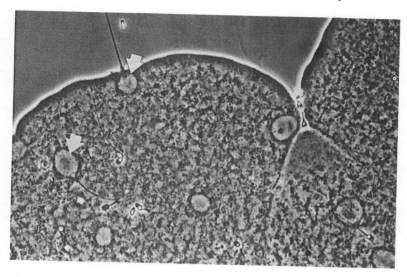

Figure 8.4 penetration of a zona-free hamster oocyte by human spermatozoa. Arrows indicate spermatozoa which have penetrated the ovum and are beginning to swell as the sperm nucleus decondenses

into account the time course of the process and the sequence of events involved. The term fertilization covers a wide range of events, beginning with the passage of the spermatozoon through the dense cloud of cumulus cells that surround the ovum and ending in cytokinesis, i.e. the division of the oocyte into two cells. Although the whole process lasts about twenty-four hours, many of the events which are targeted by contraceptive vaccines occur during the earliest stages of fertilization. To find out whether a particular antibody has succeeded in disrupting the fertilization of the human ovum, we would need to grow the zygote in culture only as far as the pronuclear stage of development, which is reached about fifteen hours after the ovum has been exposed to the spermatozoa. At this stage of fertilization the spermatozoon has succeeded in crossing the zona pellucida and fusing with the vitelline membrane of the oocyte, i.e. it has successfully accomplished both of the recognition events which gamete-based vaccines are designed to inhibit. At the pronuclear stage of development, however, the chromosomes of the spermatozoon and oocyte have not united, and the cell is still functioning on the maternal early genetic material (messenger RNA) produced during oocyte formation.

Embryonic antigens and the maternal recognition of pregnancy

Specific antigens secreted by the early conceptus or appearing on its surface could provide a further opportunity for contraceptive intervention. In general, however, the risk of abortion in the first trimester if this kind of immunization fails has limited the enthusiasm with which this approach has been pursued (Anderson and Alexander 1983). The only placental product which has been closely studied with this approach in mind is human chorionic gonadotropin (hCG) (Thanavala, Hay, and Roitt 1984). This hormone is produced by the embryonic trophoblast within seven days of fertilization and it signals the presence of the embryo to the maternal endocrine system. As a consequence, the corpus luteum of the ovary is maintained, and its continued secretion of progesterone inhibits menstruation and maintains the uterine environment for implantation of the fertilized oocyte. Immunization should neutralize this embryonic signal and lead to a series of normal or slightly extended menstrual cycles during which any pregnancy that developed would be terminated at the blastocyst stage.

A vaccine incorporating a unique amino acid sequence from the β subunit of hCG is now being assessed in clinical trials conducted under the auspices of the World Health Organisation. Research on human embryos was not required to bring this approach to fruition, because hCG continues to be produced after the blastocyst has implanted, reaching a peak at about the tenth week of pregnancy. As a result, sufficient quantities of this material could be isolated from blood samples taken in the first trimester to permit protein purification and sequencing studies. But a large number of other antigens may be expressed only transiently during the preimplantation stages of human development and, for this reason, may be more suitable for vaccine production than hCG itself. Evolving a strategy for identifying, purifying, and sequencing such antigens is, however, fraught with logistical problems related to the supply of material. It would not be possible to isolate enough antigen from human blastocysts produced by *in vitro* fertilization. A solution may be to use human teratocarcinoma cell lines which are known to possess antigens that are shared by both human embryonic tissue and cancer cells – the oncofoetal antigens. Some information could be gained about the distribution and possible function of these antigens by observing the effects of antibodies applied to the human embryo *in vitro*, but such a system would not be effective in identifying antibodies with a capacity to block the interactions between the blastocyst and endometrium – a recognition event which is similar in many ways to the sperm–oocyte interaction targeted by the gamete-oriented vaccines. To determine whether these antibodies had contraceptive potential, it would be necessary to identify an animal model in which the blastocyst expressed cross-reactive determinants.

Concluding comments

The development of new approaches to contraception is a strategically important area of research and is arguably more important than the treatment of infertility. World population continues to rise at a rate of over 400000 per day, and unwanted pregnancies continue at a very high level – for example 127000 pregnancies were electively terminated in England and Wales in 1983. The figures for IVF/ET pale into insignificance against these figures. By the end of 1985, about 10000 embryos will have been produced in the world by *in vitro* fertilization and about 1000 'test-tube' babies will have been born. Perhaps 200–500 eggs will have been donated for research designed to improve *in vitro* fertilization or study the development of congenital abnormalities, or do both of these. None of the donated eggs, to our knowledge, have been used for studies directly related to contraception. The technique of *in vitro* fertilization, however, certainly provides a potentially important and fundamentally new step for evaluating the mechanism of action and the safety of new approaches to contraception.

Much of this work need provide no ethical dilemma. The various tests that have been developed for measuring sperm function *in vitro*, including the interspecies fertilization test, allow the study of sperm function to go a long way before one needs to contemplate the fertilization of the human oocyte. By comparison, the female gamete is a very scarce resource and is going to remain so for the foreseeable future. It might be possible, with current medical resources, to collect a few thousand eggs per year for purposes of research, but their use would then be very much a question of priorities. Should contraception rank higher than the treatment of infertility or than the diagnosis and prevention of congenital defects and inherited diseases? The answer depends on one's own personal experiences, and one's views of what constitutes life. Certainly, there are no grounds for using human embryos in routine toxicological screening.

The experimental production of an embryo, as a consequence of research, does raise an ethical dilemma, but in part this could be resolved if we defined more precisely what constitutes fertilization. Stopping development at the pronuclear stage would allow many studies, although at this stage fertilization is clearly incomplete, and biochemically the cell is still functioning on maternal mRNA produced during the growth of the oocyte. Much more fundamental information would be available, of course, if the embryo were allowed to proceed through three or four cell divisions. This would allow the embryo to be karyotyped and its normality or otherwise determined (Angell *et al*. 1983). Human embryos are apparently very prone to abnormal development – and this could account for the very high loss of embryos observed before implantation. The limiting factor, in many respects, will be the willingness of women to donate oocytes for purposes of research. Studies on the attitudes of women of reproductive age in Edinburgh have shown, contrary to what public debate may have indicated, that over 75 per cent of women feel they should have a right to donate eggs for research, and more than one in five have indicated that they would wish to do so if the opportunity arose (Alder *et al*. 1986).

References

Ada, G.L., Basten, A., and Jones, W.R. (1985) Prospects for developing vaccines to control fertility. *Nature* 317: 288–89

Aitken, R.J. (1982) The contraceptive potential of anti-sperm antibodies. In S.L. Jeffcoate and M. Sandler (eds) *Progress Towards a Male Contraceptive*. Chichester: Wiley, pp. 109–34

Aitken, R.J., Richardson, D.W., and Hulme, M.J. (1984) Immunological interference with the properties of the zona pellucida. In D.B. Crighton (ed) *Immunological Aspects of Reproduction in Mammals*. London: Butterworths, pp. 305–25

Aitken, R.J., Templeton, A., Schats, R., et al. (1983) Methods for assessing the functional capacity of human spermatozoa; their role in the selection of patients for *in vitro* fertilization. In H.M. Beier and H.R. Lindner (eds) *Fertilization of the Human Egg In Vitro: Biological Basis and Clinical Applications*. Berlin: Springer-Verlag, pp. 147–65

Alder, E.A., Baird, D.T., Lees, M., Lincoln, D., Loudon, N., and Templeton, A.A. (1986) Attitudes of women of reproductive age to *in vitro* fertilisation (IVF) and embryo research. *Journal of Biosocial Science*, submitted

Anderson, D.J. and Alexander, N.J. (1983) A new look at antifertility vaccines. *Fertility and Sterility* 40: 557–71

Angell, R.R., Aitken, R.J., Van Look, P.F.A., Lumsden, M.A., and Templeton, A.A. (1983) Chromosome abnormalities in human embryos after *in vitro* fertilization. *Nature* 303: 336–38

Dor, J., Rudak, E.A., and Aitken, R.J. (1981) Anti-sperm antibodies: their effect on the process of fertilization studied *in vitro*. *Fertility and Sterility* 35: 535–41

Fong, H.H.S. (1984) Current status of gossypol, zoapatanol, and other plant-derived fertility regulating agents. In P. Krogsgaard-Larsen *et al*. (eds) *Natural Products and Drug Development*. Copenhagen: Munksgaard (Alfred Benzon Symposium 20), pp. 355–73

Graham, S. and Fraser, I.S. (1982) The progestogen-only mini-pill. *Contraception* 26: 373–88

Healy, D.L. and Fraser, H.M. (1985) The antiprogesterones are coming: menses induction, abortion and labour? *British Medical Journal* 290: 580–81

Thanavala, Y.M., Hay, F.C., and Roitt, I.M. (1984) Fertility control by immunization against hCG. In D.B. Crighton (ed.) *Immunological Aspects of Reproduction in Mammals*. London: Butterworths, pp. 327–44

Yanagimachi, R., Yanagimachi, H., and Rogers, B.J. (1976) The use of zona free animal ova as a test system for the assessment of the fertilizing capacity of human spermatozoa. *Biology of Reproduction* 15: 471–76

Yanagimachi, R., Lopata, A., Odom, C.B., Bronson, R.A., Mahi, L.A., and Nicolson, G.L. (1979) Retention of biological characteristics of zona pellucida in highly concentrated salt solution: the use of salt stored eggs for assessing the fertilizing capacity of spermatozoa. *Fertility and Sterility* 31: 562–74

Discussion

Harper: Many of the genes which have been cloned in humans have been detected as a result of partial homology with gene products in other species. With these key processes in early development many of the genes are likely to be very highly conserved between species. You mentioned that the human zona pellucida was very difficult to work with, but rather than using pig genes directly wouldn't it be more logical to use pig genes to clone the human gene and thus get a specific human gene? Also, in terms of identifying some of the structural abnormalities in human development, won't some of the candidate genes be understood much better from early experimental work on animals? One could then look across to their counterparts in humans in order to identify the specific human genes involved in developmental defects.

Aitken: The use of porcine zonae pellucidae antigens as the raw material for engineering a vaccine has some advantages. For instance, it will be immunogenic in the human and the antibodies it elicits are known to inhibit the fertilization of human ova *in vitro*. It might well be possible to use the porcine antigen as a means of probing the complementary gene for the human zona pellucida. These two approaches are not mutually exclusive. There are people working on both areas and only time will tell which is more effective.

Williamson: The two are complementary and the use of animal models for studying normal development is a very legitimate and useful technique, which only occasionally leads us astray. The use of animals for the study of abnormal hereditary conditions is much less likely to be useful. Laboratory animals are very standardized and homogeneous, whereas most humans live in outbred populations with different pathological determinants from those of the inbred animals used in laboratories.

Weatherall: Once you have defined regulatory genes in animal models, if you want to understand anything about human development you will have to develop probes to determine at what stage of development those genes are activated.

Harper: I don't doubt that. I was just wondering whether the degree of homology wasn't such that this might be a better way to go, in some instances, than using a blind mapping technique in human families.

Maddox: Would that not be a fair point for an ethical committee or a regulatory committee to decide on, allowing you to do the first part of your experiments while acknowledging that ultimately you may have to have human embryos?

Clothier: If it is justifiable at all, why is it not justifiable from the beginning?

Maddox: There is the practical question of getting the oocytes. There is some very small risk to the women concerned.

McLaren: In the early days of thinking about contraceptive vaccines the idea was put forward that there was a possible risk in using an antigen which was present all the time in the body of the woman or the man. Sperm are always present in a man's body and the zona pellucida is always present in a woman's body. If this idea is valid, a protein produced by the very early cleavage stage would be a particularly suitable target for contraception because it would do away with that risk. Is that a hazard that is still recognized or has it been forgotten about?

Aitken: It hasn't been entirely forgotten. A recent report in *Nature* (Ada, Basten, and Jones 1985) suggested that the ideal target would be an antigen which is expressed transiently, as you are suggesting, or in small amounts. With the zona pellucida, for example, a very small amount of material is present within the ovary. The antigens of which this structure is composed never escape into the peripheral circulation so there would be no danger of immune complex diseases. Furthermore, antibodies raised against the zona pellucida are extremely specific; they will not cross-react with any other tissue in the body. Similarly, if you are going to immunize against sperm antigens the most logical target is the woman rather than the man. In men only about 5 per cent of circulating immunoglobulin G (IgG) ever finds its way into the seminal plasma, so the induction of systemic immunity is unlikely to result in an adequate exposure of the spermatozoa to the appropriate antibodies. In women, however, sperm antigens exhibit a transient presence and are accessible to circulating antibodies.

Weatherall:　There is no immediate need for research on developmental genetics in early human embryos. What we are desperately worried about is closing the door in the long term. Once we have got the information from animal models we cannot approach pathological development in humans without some work on human material.

McLaren:　I would say that it isn't ethical even to use more animal material than is essential for research. I wouldn't want to use human material if I could use animal material, and I wouldn't want to use later stages of human development if I could use earlier stages for the same result.

Clothier:　Is that because you have an instinctive objection to using human material even though it is justified by the benefits to be obtained?

McLaren:　In research on either animal or human material one would want to use the least amount that would effectively get the results. The logic of that is based on the sanctity of life. This view has been put forward by various ethicists here but it is shared by scientists: life is not to be squandered pointlessly. That is ethical rather than logical, I suppose.

Hull:　We are perhaps succumbing to the widespread assumption that our choice of experimental material is based on accepting the lesser of two evils. That philosophy certainly applies to the termination of pregnancy but I don't believe it applies to experimentation on the early embryo. I would not accept that it is the lesser of two evils. I see no evil in it at all.

Clothier: That is what prompted me to ask why it is not justifiable from the beginning.

McLaren: But we are working in a society where certain activities are unacceptable to a certain number of people. We have to take that into account.

Clothier: So you do as little as possible out of respect for the feelings of society?

Hull: We must take society into account but society makes the general assumption that abortion is clearly the lesser of two evils and that embryo research simply represents one end of the same process, the thin end of the wedge. I don't believe it is part of the same continuum at all.

Dunstan: Instead of the lesser of two evils as a formula would you prefer the least drastic remedy, Dr Hull? That would be consistent with preferring to work on tissues rather than whole animals, and on animals rather than humans.

Edwards: It would imply that one would have to be prepared to go to the most drastic remedy if it were necessary.

Dunstan: But the principle is to choose the least drastic one first.

Clothier: On the other hand it may be drastic but justifiable.

Hull: This still seems to imply that there is something evil about experimenting on early embryos. I don't believe it is evil at all.

McLaren: I don't think it is evil but I do think that the material is very precious.

Clothier: Precious in the sense that it is different from all other living material because it is human?

McLaren: It is precious because it has been donated.

Clothier: That is a switch of ground altogether.

Baird: Professor Dunstan put it well at another meeting here when he said that the presumption in most societies is in favour of life (Dunstan 1985, p. 115). The life of the conceptus, embryo, foetus, and infant has to be preserved but there are circumstances in which that right can be overridden. The onus all the time, from a two-cell embryo onwards, is to demonstrate that there is good cause to override that right.

Clothier: That is, the end will justify the means, although that is a bad way of saying this.

Williamson: I agree with the way David Baird has put it. Anne McLaren's points about public unease and the scarcity of this material are true but are a different order of argument. I don't think it is a question of the end justifying the means but rather one of alternatives. There are alternative outcomes and each of us chooses between them in terms of our perception of their advantages and disadvantages, rather than in absolute terms.

Clothier: Many of us believe it is right to fight a war in defence of freedom, or to shoot an assailant in order to protect your own life or the lives of those very close to you. The law has always recognized that.

References

Ada, G.L., Basten, A., and Jones, W.R. (1985) Prospects for developing vaccines to control fertility. *Nature* 317: 288–89

Dunstan, G.R. (1985) In *Abortion: Medical Progress and Social Implications*. Pitman, London (Ciba Foundation Symposium 115) p. 115

NINE

Status of the pre-embryo (general discussion)

Braude: May I raise a point about the special status of the human pre-embryo, or whatever you wish to call it? There is an overall feeling that this group of cells *in vitro* is special because it has the potential of forming a human being or person. In reality this potential is relative, for it changes with the developmental stage. As the fertilized egg cleaves through to the blastocyst stage, it has an increased possibility of becoming a person if it is replaced into a suitably receptive uterus. However, a few days later, once the blastocyst has hatched from its zona pellucida, it will not implant even if it is transferred to a uterus. Thus, despite being developmentally more advanced, perhaps even as much as ten or fourteen days after fertilization, that blastocyst has missed the narrow window for successful implantation and now has absolutely no potential to form a person. I would like to know, then, what is the moral status of this embryonic 'non-person'?

Edwards: When we do research on embryos or observe embryos we ask our patients for permission to do research but we do not specify the nature of the research. I am not sure whether the patients can give informed consent to detailed proposals. By asking them to consent, we make the assumption that the embryos belong to the adults. Is it necessary to ask for consent to a detailed piece of work once the embryos are *in vitro*, or is consent to a general request enough?

Clothier: If an embryo is donated for research it is clearly an outright gift and the person to whom it is given can use it as he or she thinks proper. If embryos are taken for therapeutic reasons the donor has not necessarily parted with them until after two or three have been selected for implantation, after which I suppose you ask the person if they want to donate the surplus for research. If the donor says yes, the property immediately passes from that person to you. If the donor asks for the surplus oocytes to be destroyed you would destroy them because you recognize that that person has a proprietary right in them. After all, we have proprietary rights in other tissues and organs of our bodies.

Edwards: If we ask the parents for consent this implies that the embryo belongs to the adult and has no rights of its own.

Clothier: At that point it would still be possible to return it to the owner, improved by fertilization. That is why they lent it to you in the first place, so that it might be worked upon and returned in a better state.

Edwards: But what about those donated for research?

Clothier: The limitations on their use would be ethical. There may be legal limitations but the donor has abandoned them and no longer has any rights in them.

Gerard: One can make donations so long as it is a chattel that one is donating.

Edwards: Can you donate children? Are they chattels, and, if not, at what embryonic stage do they lose this status?

Gerard: No, you can't have ownership rights in a living human being, though the law recognizes a limited right of possession of a human body after death, with the corresponding obligation to dispose of that body. These concepts, which now apply to the period after life, might be adapted to regulate the use of embryos during a period before life.

Clothier: Children have a separate existence, haven't they?

Gerard: Another point that worries me is whose consent are we talking about? Professor Edwards speaks of the mother only; but if we are talking about an embryo or a pre-embryo, a fertilized thing, who represents that thing – the mother or the father or neither? Who has authority to consent on its behalf?

Clothier: We all recognize there is a difference between this elementary cluster of cells and a life in being, as the law used to call it. There is perhaps a difference between not being able to possess another human being or a life in being, and being able to possess and part with a cluster of cells.

Rights or duties?

Baird: Does the foetus of less than twenty-eight weeks have any legal rights?

Clothier: It is protected by the Infant Life Preservation Act 1929. It has the right to be allowed to continue to develop and to live.

Baird: That is overriden by the 1967 Abortion Act.

Clothier: Only in cases where the law prescribes.

Dunstan: We may be approaching this question about status on the wrong grounds. I would protect the embryo in terms of our *duties* towards it, because I cannot recognize in law any *rights* for a foetus or an embryo until we start protecting it by law. We have duties to the foetus long before it secures a new sort of protection under the Infant Life Preservation Act.

Edwards: I am not clear what you mean about one's duty to the embryo, Professor Dunstan. Does Peter Braude owe a greater duty to the parthenogenetic embryo in alcohol than to the one he actually establishes *in vitro* or even *in vivo*?

Dunstan: One of the questions I had stored up was what is the future of the embryos that are stored? I can't answer anything until I know more about it. In general there are many important areas of life where we have duties which are not grounded in rights – towards animals for instance; or to someone outside in a violent thunderstorm who has no right of entry into my home: I have a duty to offer that person shelter. We do great disservice to the whole process of discussion in society if we invent rights for everything. Let us stick to duties and see how far we can go. In our long history, duties to the unborn child have been acknowledged and enforced but there has never been a word about rights.

Rodeck: I am much in favour of that because it implies *responsibility* whereas 'rights' create expectations and demands and can diminish a sense of responsibility or duty. We also need a much more sophisticated and educated public to realize that doctors and scientists are not omniscient. Many things that we do require experimentation. For example, we need ethical clinical controlled trials to compare one method of treatment with another, and this requires patients who regard it as a duty to society to participate.

Ethics of experimentation

Casey: With any regulatory regime there is the possibility that experiments will be done elsewhere which are ruled illegitimate under that regime. To what extent is it ethical to use the results of those experiments? The question would arise in this case if the Powell Bill (the Unborn Children [Protection] Bill) were passed and if advances were made in Australia which it was then proposed to use in clinical practice in the UK. It must occur in other areas of science. The concentration camp experiments in World War II clearly transgressed what is normally acceptable but they produced results which would otherwise be considered scientifically valid. There may be other examples involving the unacceptable use of animals, for instance. How do scientists feel about that?

Clothier: Have such experimental results been put into effect here?

Casey: According to a piece in *New Scientist* (Dixon 1985) the concentration camp experiments are in some sense regarded as definitive on the cooling of human bodies in water. Some experimenters have avoided using them; others have used them and quoted them as scientific references but not made any acknowledgement of the fact that they were obtained under unacceptable circumstances.

Clothier: Wouldn't doctors whose duty is to relieve suffering or cure patients feel great difficulty about not using some technique which they had heard of and which was almost certain to cure their patients, however much they deplored the manner in which that knowledge had been gained? Once it is gained it is there for use on patients.

Braude: We were faced with this in the Anatomy Department in Cambridge. I don't know how it got there but there is a roll of film showing the movement of bones in the upper limb which was obtained by X-ray cinematography of victims in a German concentration camp. We had to decide whether to show this film to the medical students to demonstrate to them what happens anatomically, or to deny access because of the methods used to make the film. We decided it would be disrespectful not to use the film, for people had obviously suffered and indeed died as a result of this work, but the information now stood. It should never have been made but the information provided is unique.

Clothier: If the knowledge can only be imparted effectively that way, that may be a justifiable decision. It is not such a strong case as applying a treatment that you have learnt of from abroad.

Baird: A medical person might use the knowledge but the second question you asked was would somebody who held an ethical objection to experimenting on embryos be justified in benefiting from the knowledge obtained from such experiments.

Maddox: It is like the question of whether non-members of a trades union should benefit from the results of wage negotiations.

Hull: Or that we should not be prepared to learn any lessons from history.

Iglesias: Morality has to do with the way we treat one another, and with what we choose to do in a particular case. Where results have been obtained from experiments of that kind, the choice of using the knowledge provided by those results is not evil in itself. Yet if one co-operated in some way in establishing those results that would be a different question.

Dr Edwards raised a question about law and morality. Moral values cannot be discerned according to how many people say something is right or wrong. Acceptability by most people does not make a practice right – counting heads is not a way to determine good and evil. At the same time the law has to be sensitive to what is going on and what society thinks, but without abandoning principles of natural justice.

Harper: The question about benefit from research elsewhere is slightly different from where something unethical has been done in the past that we may now benefit from. The question is really whether it is right to frame a law to make something illegal while assuming that what we are making illegal will be done elsewhere and we shall thereby benefit from it. That is very definitely not ethical whereas some of these other cases are much harder to argue.

Bowker: That might become very explicit and real. There is no international morality and if you have a very different anthropology (i.e. a different understanding of what human nature is) this does become problematic. Professor Dunstan spoke about duties. Hinduism would totally agree that what you have to focus on is *dharma*, or the duty of a doctor at a particular time, without necessarily any reference to abstract concepts like 'person'. A whole medical society might do things which would be abhorrent to another anthropology. This is by no means confined to a concentration camp syndrome. If you are a doctor with *dharma* or duties and you have to be reborn eight-four million times, eventually you will see that perhaps you would not now act in the way that *was* appropriate as you move towards *moksha* (release). The Jains are the most specific about this, but they are a rather small community. They have applied the toleration of others involved in the killing of animals to medical research.

Social judgements

Dyson: Theologians and philosophers regard experimentation principally as a good, just as we regard human life as a good. The problem is the conflict between the two and how to handle this conflict. I suggest that a statement that something is a human person is not wholly a factual statement although it includes factual elements. Like aesthetic judgements, statements of this kind include factual components and evaluative components. When I say something is a person I am making an evaluation which cannot be wholly grounded in fact, but is also based on intuition or common sentiment or something of that kind. I would be very hesitant to say that an artificially fertilized ovum is in the same category as a normal embryo in the uterus. I would not want to make the same evaluative judgement about that as about normal development.

Because we are dealing here with language which is a combination of facts and values, we need to listen to society very carefully. In the community there are not only prejudices and negative views but also positive inherited perceptions of values and how to handle clashes of values. It seems to me that on the question of research you are not allowing some of these conflicts of value to come out, but we have to work through them. That is what we are looking for at the moment.

I don't altogether agree with the view that the Voluntary Licensing Authority [set up jointly by the Royal College of Obstetricians and Gynaecologists and the Medical Research Council to function along the lines of the Statutory Licensing Authority recommended by the Warnock Committee] can deal with this. Where is that body to get its general principles from? It can't settle each case as it comes up without appealing to general principles. We need more dialogue between society and scientists in which we try to work out some middle-range principles. Sometimes these will come into conflict and we want to know what the limiting factors would be. We need to generate some sense of these middle-range questions. We have to recognize both the factual questions, the ways in which the prejudices and misunderstandings of society have to be corrected, and the inherited but revisable moral perceptions of society on how one can treat children, what kind of experiments are legitimate, what kind of consensus is required, and so on.

Braude: That is a strong argument. The Warnock Committee handled this very well in putting forward the fourteen-day rule that was without doubt a compromise between the scientific community and what the public would be prepared to accept. What worries me is that sometimes what society is prepared to accept, and what it puts forward, is based on a dogma that has now been challenged by new technology.

Dyson: That was why I said we would have to make reciprocally generated judgements and evaluations. I agree with you, but the fourteen-day rule is problematic. I see Warnock as having reported at a time when the kind of dialogue and debate I have just described had not yet been adequately undertaken. Until that happens we are going to have very arbitrary guidelines. When some sort of middle-range principles find a reasonably common acceptance, revisions will have to take place. We haven't reached the position yet in which these middle-range principles have been reciprocally teased out and understood.

Rodeck: On most of these issues we don't really know what society thinks or wants. The Warnock Report, for example, was the result of the views of members of the committee, and advice and information obtained from various bodies (Warnock 1984). This is a highly selected group and does not necessarily represent what the majority of people in the UK would want or think about those questions. There have indeed been very few surveys on the opinions of ordinary people, but one of the daily national newspapers had an article recently about an American survey. About 80 per cent of people were in favour of this kind of work if it was used to prevent handicap, for example.

Baird: In the Edinburgh area, as Dr Aitken mentioned in his paper, we surveyed over 1000 women attending a family planning clinic, over 500 attending an antenatal clinic, and a smaller number attending the infertility clinic (see Alder *et al.* 1986). About 12 per cent were Catholics. The results in the three groups were almost identical. Just under 10 per cent were totally opposed to any form of research on embryos, no matter what the objective, but between 60 and 70 per cent were in favour of research on human embryos up to fourteen days, if the objectives were either to improve *in vitro* fertilization techniques or to get greater knowledge of the causes of congenital abnormalities. That is one segment of a population in one area of the country, and all the women were in the reproductive age group so they may not be representative of the whole population – but they are in an age group to which these techniques have most application.

Clothier: The Warnock Committee advertised for evidence from interested parties. The Report (Warnock 1984) has a long list of organizations and individuals who gave evidence.

Baird: But over 99 per cent of the population do not submit evidence to such committees.

Edwards: Asking society to comment is notoriously unreliable. I am sure that if there was a television programme which raised any alarm about a procedure, then 95 per cent of your sample in Edinburgh might vote the other way. Anna Southam pointed out years ago that many doctors did not accept abortion until the law was changed (Southam and Driver 1973). They changed their minds after the law was changed.

Embryo or pre-embryo?

Clothier: The expression pre-embryo was originally suggested by Dr Penelope Leach, who is also a member of the Voluntary Licensing Authority. The connotation in the minds of the public is that the embryo already has recognizable human characteristics, whereas what we were talking about could not be said to have human characteristics. 'Conceptus' connotes the creation of a new life in being, so we arrived at 'pre-embryo'. It would be useful to know what you think of this word.

Maddox: I think it is a cosmetic trick.

McLaren: There is ambiguity in the way scientists use the term 'embryo', as I said earlier (Chapter 2), and we are not justified in continuing to use the term embryo in both senses. We are not talking about cosmetics but about clarity.

Maddox: In the past three years the general public has heard so much about embryos that if scientists now try to say that pre-embryos are what you are concerned with, people would be rather offended. In public discussion it seems to me proper to use the term in two senses without differentiating.

Edwards: The embryo means something much later to doctors than it does to scientists. I am not sure what scientists or doctors would think about 'pre-embryo', but many would question it. In a sense, of course, it is almost an abbreviation of 'preimplantation embryo'. Why can't we stick to the terms we have used for many years, such as preimplantation embryos, morulae, blastocysts, and implanted embryos? This is my opinion, but if a new term clarifies matters, it should perhaps be considered seriously.

Clothier: We all thought that 'pre-embryo' did clarify matters.

References

Alder, E.M., Baird, D.T., Lees, M.M., Lincoln, D., Loudon, N., and Templeton, A.A. (1986) Attitudes of women of reproductive age to *in vitro* fertilization and embryo research. *Journal of Biosocial Science*, submitted.

Dixon, B. (1985) Citations of shame. *New Scientist* No. 1445: 31 (28 February)

Southam, A. and Driver, E.D. (1973) Biomedical, social, and legal implications of fertility control. In E.S.E. Hafez and T.N. Evans (eds) *Human Reproduction, Conception and Contraception.* Hagerstown, MD: Harper & Row

Warnock, M. (Chairman) (1984) *Report of the Committee of Inquiry into Human Fertilisation and Embryology.* London: HMSO (Department of Health & Social Security) Cmnd. 9314

TEN

The sociology of 'public morality'

G. Hawthorn

Opinion polls show a majority of the population in the United Kingdom to be against Enoch Powell's Bill for the Protection of the Unborn Child. The possibility that this is one more instance of a growing 'liberalization' of attitude is questioned. It can be seen as an enduring and comprehensible conservatism. Nevertheless, it is not the conservatism reflected either in the Bill or in discussions of a 'common public morality'. On many issues, including the new techniques of fertilization, there may be no such morality and, accordingly, no authority to impose it. The Warnock Committee's discussion of these issues, whatever one may think of the conclusions to which it comes, is inadequate.

Public opinion on *in vitro* fertilization and embryo research

On the 28, 29, and 30 June, 1985, National Opinion Polls telephoned a sample of 1017 people in the UK to find out whether the Private Member's Bill introduced in Parliament by Enoch Powell (1985) had their support. NOP's first question was:

> To enable some women to become pregnant, doctors can fertilize eggs outside the womb and then replace the embryo in the womb for the rest of pregnancy. Doctors normally grow several embryos and use

just one, discarding those they don't use. Some people think that it's morally wrong to do this, but others say it's necessary to grow more embryos than are used to increase the chance of a successful pregnancy. Which of these views is closer to your own, or haven't you thought about it enough to say?

The answers given are in Table 10.1.

Second, NOP asked whether embryos that had been grown but not implanted should be used 'for research on genetic diseases and birth handicaps'. Powell wants to prohibit this. But only a quarter of the sample agreed with him; a half definitely did not. Finally, NOP asked:

Doctors also use human embryos in research work to improve their knowledge of the cause of disease and handicap in newly-born children. Do you approve or disapprove of human embryos being used in this way, or haven't you thought about it enough to say?

The answers are in Table 10.2.

Table 10.1   Attitudes to *in vitro* fertilization

		age (years)						
	all	15–24	25–34	35–54	55–64	65 +	male	female
base:	1017	193	173	315	153	183	478	539
	%	%	%	%	%	%	%	%
morally wrong	28	16	20	33	34	37	26	30
necessary	49	55	59	49	42	37	52	46
not thought	23	29	21	18	24	26	22	24

Table 10.2   Attitudes to using embryos in medical research

		age (years)						
	all	15–24	25–34	35–54	55–64	65 +	male	female
base:	1017	193	173	315	153	183	478	539
	%	%	%	%	%	%	%	%
approve	52	52	54	54	56	40	57	48
disapprove	26	22	23	28	27	31	24	28
not thought	22	21	23	18	17	29	19	24

Polls are only ever indicative. The vicissitudes of sampling, the unknown effects of surrounding circumstance, the way in which the questions are worded and actually asked, and, not least, the possibility that those polled are prompted into having a view they had not come to before, all counsel caution. Nevertheless, respondents on this occasion were allowed 'not to have thought enough' about the issue, and the results are clear. About half of them supported present practices; of those who didn't, more were over 65, and more were women.

In trying to explain these findings, one can pursue the various distinctions and try to discern the differences of opinion not only by age and sex but also by education, or occupation, or religion, or ethnic group, or some other such factor. No doubt there are such differences; they certainly appear in more elaborate surveys on other issues. There is, however, another explanatory strategy. This − longitudinal rather than cross-sectional − is to look for differences over time. Often, as in this poll, there is information only on age. Accordingly, to decide whether what the NOP reveals of the greater nervousness about the new techniques in the older respondents is an effect of age itself, or an effect of generation, one would have to have evidence on these people's attitudes when they were young. Where this evidence is available, for example on people's political preferences measured by their votes at successive elections, it suggests that the effects of generation are strong. No such information is available on attitudes towards intervening in reproduction. But the variation in Tables 10.1 and 10.2 is at least consistent with the widely-held presumption that attitudes towards such interventions have been becoming more 'liberal'.

This presumption, though, may be wrong. Consider the case of attitudes towards the availability of abortion. Marsh and Calderbank (1985) have re-analysed the results of some of the relevant polls on this issue since 1969 and found a remarkable stability of view. Their re-analysis does, as they say, suggest a paradox. Those who think the law ought not to be changed to make abortion easier to obtain have consistently outnumbered by a quarter those who think it should be changed. Yet those who think that abortion should be readily available have equally consistently outnumbered those who think it never should. But the paradox can perhaps be resolved by the fact that since the early 1970s the law in England, Scotland, and Wales has been moderately permissive. The wording of the questions may also play some part. But it is striking that there is no statistically significant variation over time in the proportions going one way or another within each of these series. Opinion on the availability of abortion, if opinion polls measure it, is remarkably stable. This is supported by other polls on analogous issues.

It does not yet make sense to ask how stable opinions on the new techniques of fertilization are. But if they should turn out to be as stable as those on abortion, the apparent contrast in direction between the two – between the relative liberality of those on the one side and the relative conservatism of those on the other – may not be a contrast at all. Abortion interferes to arrest reproduction; the new techniques of fertilization interfere to facilitate it. One is against the normal course of events; the other is not. In each case, the opinions picked up by the polls are, unsurprisingly, opinions in favour of normality, and in this sense conservative.

Private, public, and common morality

Nevertheless, if opinions on these more 'private' matters do resemble each other, they nevertheless differ from opinions on more obviously 'public' ones. As Marsh and Calderbank (1985) point out, mentioning the instance of attitudes over the past twenty years to our membership of the EEC, opinions on the latter are much less steady, much more likely to vary over time. But there is more than this to say about the distinction between the public and the private, and about a third category, the 'common', that runs across each and in its frequent use has thus confused both.

Twenty years or so ago, there was a celebrated exchange between Hart and Devlin on the relation between the law and morality (Hart 1963; Devlin 1965). 'The issue', as Devlin put it, was 'whether there is a realm of private morality and immorality that is not the law's business.' Hart claimed that there was such a realm. He argued, like J.S. Mill before him, that an act is only of public concern if practically it threatens some person or set of persons who are not party to it. Then, and only then, should the law intercede, but it should do so only to protect. Devlin disagreed. He suggested that 'there is general agreement' that Hart's doctrine 'is not enough, that the law should prevent a man from, for example, corrupting the morals of youth or offending the moral standards of others by a public display of what they regard as vice'. And the law, he concluded, 'cannot interfere in these ways except from the basis of a common or public morality'.

Devlin had no doubt that it should so interfere because he had no doubt that there was such a morality, 'a blend of custom and conviction', in Rostow's description, 'of reason and feeling, of experience and prejudice'. Moreover, since this is a democracy, and since, Devlin believed, 'there is no pressure whatever – the sort of pressure that governments have to take account of sooner or later – for any reform of the law based on the extrusion of moral principle', since 'Mill's doctrine of liberty has made', as he put it, 'no conquests on *terra firma*', the law had to recognize it. An educated man, he added, who dislikes such a conclusion, who is 'armed only with reason' and 'disdainful of custom and strength of feeling', 'had better not venture outside his academy, for if he does, he will have to deal with forces he cannot understand'.

Devlin, but not Hart, thus ran together 'public' and 'common' morality and justified its enactment in the law. Indeed, Devlin was quite clear that the realm of truly 'private' morality was limited, even negligible. But the three categories have to be much more carefully distinguished. At one extreme, as Devlin implies, the realm of 'private' morality may indeed be limited. It may only extend to those acts performed by individuals or very small numbers of individuals in circumstances, usually domestic, in which other people not only may not be affected by them but may never even hear about them. The new techniques of fertilization are an instance. At the other extreme, there are 'public' acts which in themselves or in their consequences unavoidably affect other people, perhaps a majority of other people. A 'common' morality, however, may be either of these or both or a third thing, rather different from each. It may be a morality subscribed to by most people, even all, and applied to acts that are, in the sense I have just suggested, 'private'. It may be a 'public' morality. Or it may be a morality which is neither 'private' nor 'public' in the commonsensical senses I have distinguished, but is 'common' or 'communal' in the different and much stronger sense that it is, or is part of, what constitutes the community as it is, so that to violate this morality is to violate or otherwise undermine the community *as that community.*

These distinctions are difficult to draw and sustain; it is not surprising that they are so often run together. Thus, at the start of its report, the Warnock Committee itself suggests that 'The law itself, binding on everyone in society, whatever their beliefs, is the embodiment of a common moral position' (Warnock 1984, Foreword, para. 6). Weakly, this can be interpreted to mean that there is a common morality in the sense that most individuals subscribe to a 'public' morality, enshrined in the law, which defines the limits of any 'private' morality 'whatever', as Warnock says, that private morality may be. More strongly, it could be interpreted to mean that there is a 'common' morality, the observance of which is what makes the community or society the community or society it is; and that the law for that community exists to maintain it, 'whatever' else individuals in that community may or may not happen to believe.

The difference between the two interpretations is clearly brought out by MacIntyre. He considers most people in Britain to be in favour of 'a pragmatic approach to problems, co-operativeness, fair play, tolerance [and] a gift for compromise' (MacIntyre 1967). These, he says, are secondary virtues. 'Secondary virtues concern the way in which we should go about our projects; their cultivation will not assist us in discovering upon which projects we ought to be engaged.' There is no longer any agreement in Britain about these ends, about 'primary' virtues. 'The extent to which different moral criteria are established in common amongst us is extremely uncertain, and therefore the kind of appeal that we are able to make when we use moral predicates is also uncertain.' We often talk as though we were a moral community, our language contains 'moral predicates' which suggest it, but this, continues MacIntyre, is 'illusion'. Not to put too fine a point on it, we rattle around, *faute de mieux*, in a residual, now merely rhetorical, Christianity. Our actual *terra firma, pace* Devlin and to MacIntyre's distress, is the one that Mill mapped out.

Thus also, although less lucidly, the Warnock Committee. Having said that the law embodies 'a common moral position', it inclines toward the weaker of the two possible interpretations of its earlier remark and claims that 'what is legally permissible may be thought of as the minimum requirement[s] for a tolerable society'. It defends the recommendations it makes by saying that the 'evidence' it received in the course of its deliberations indicates that these requirements are, in the field it is considering and in order of importance, the care and psychological health of children – 'of paramount importance', the integrity of the nuclear family, and clarity and consistency in the claims that can be reasonably made by those who have contributed to fertilization or gestation and, where they are different, those who have acted as parents.

Warnock, morality, and authority

But it might now be clear that Warnock's minimally common and so, it is supposed, legitimately public morality refers to two rather different kinds of thing: first, the interests of those – children – who may not be able to speak for themselves, and the interests of those, genitors, natural mothers, and parents, which may conflict or may come to conflict; and second, the more truly 'communal' interest, in the sense in which MacIntyre uses the word, of the integrity of the nuclear family. And in not making the distinction clear, the committee compounds rather than clarifies the corollary, the confusion about who can claim moral authority and in virtue of what.

Devlin, MacIntyre, and those who argue like them have a clear and unequivocal answer to this question. A common morality, in the strong sense, would, if it existed, be its own sufficient authority. It is all that Parliament, or the courts, or the Church, or some other such institution needs to act. There may be more or less technical arguments about how to discover what it is. But it is there to be discovered. And once it is, the institutions can confidently dictate and enforce it. They can do so because those who dispute it, or act against it, are in so doing undermining any claim they may make to equality of treatment and respect, undermining any claim they may make actually to belong.

Others answer differently. If the morality is not there to be discovered, but only to be chosen; and if people consider the act or acts in question as a 'private' matter, not of 'public' concern; then even if they all happen to agree on how, in any respect, they should act, there is not, except in the thin and trivial sense, a 'common' or 'public' morality. There can therefore be no authority for publicly imposing one course of action rather than another, unless there is reason to think that people are mis-informed about the consequences of their choice, or that, in acting on it, they will adversely affect others by more than mere offence.

That, roughly speaking, was the conclusion in 1959 of the Wolfenden Committee on Homosexual Offences and Prostitution – the conclusion which sparked off the argument between Hart and Devlin. The Warnock Committee does not go quite so far. One reason for this is clear and uncontroversial. The new techniques of fertilization have implications for what have come to be agreed to be the rights of 'parents', indivisibly understood, and children. Unlike homosexuality between consenting adults, or prosti-tution, they are private acts with public consequences. But when it considers the question of surrogacy, the Warnock Committee falters. It recognizes (Warnock 1984: 8.14) that couples have 'a perfect right to enter into such agreements if they so wish', and that they won't do so lightly, but a majority of its members concluded (8.17) that those couples may nevertheless not know their own best interests in doing so. The Committee accordingly recommends that such arrangements be proscribed. The argu-ment it offers – that if they are not proscribed people will be treating each other as means and not ends – sits uneasily with the concession of rights and of the capacity of those entering into such arrangements to know their own interests; and its more practical worries are perfectly well answered, from the analogy of adoption, by the two dissenting members. I suspect that what really decided the majority, as Warnock herself has since made clear (1985), was a reluctance to interfere with established practices just because they have been established practices, because any departure from them went against the common morality, in the strong sense in which I have used that term. The causal connection between a woman's womb and the child of that womb appears, in the committee's view, also to be a moral connection, its own best defence, and thus, its own authority (Warnock 1985).

But my concern is not with the acceptability or otherwise of Warnock's conclusions. It is with the arguments by which they are arrived at and the authority they may fairly claim. In its arguments, I do not think the Warnock Committee paid sufficient attention to the critical distinctions between private, public, and common moralities. In its recommendations, partly because of this, partly because it fails to explain what could and should count as evidence for or against morality, and partly because the establishment of such a committee, a convention of our political practice, inclines everyone to accept that there is a single best and thus authoritative view to be had, I do not think that it paid sufficient attention to the basis of the authority it presumed to be able to claim.

In all but the issue of surrogacy, this may not, in practice, matter. The recommendations run with what seems to be the conservative current of ordinary opinion. But there is irony, as well as error, in the conservatism of Powell's Bill.

Acknowledgements

I am grateful to Catherine Marsh for information on recent opinion polls and for letting me see her recent paper (Marsh and Calderbank 1985); and to Bernard Williams for his extremely helpful remarks on an earlier version of this one.

References

Devlin, P. (1965) *The Enforcement of Morals.* London: Oxford University Press

Hart, H.L.A. (1963) *Law, Liberty, and Morality.* London: Oxford University Press

MacIntyre, A. (1967) *Secularisation and Moral Change.* London: Oxford University Press

Marsh, C. and Calderbank, D. (1985) *Public Attitudes to Abortion 1967–1982: Stability and Complexity.* Mimeo (available from Social and Political Sciences Committee, Free School Lane, Cambridge, CB2 3RQ)

National Opinion Polls (1985) *Political, Social and Economic Review 54.* London: NOP

Powell, E. (1985) *Unborn Children (Protection) Bill.*

Warnock, M. (Chairman) (1984) *Report of the Committee of Inquiry into Human Fertilisation and Embryology.* London: HMSO (Department of Health & Social Security) Cmnd. 9314

Warnock, M. (1985) Legal surrogacy: not for love or money? *The Listener* 113 (2893): 2–4

Wolfenden, J. (Chairman) (1959) *Report of the Committee on Homosexual Offences and Prostitution.* London: HMSO (Home Office) Cmnd. 247

Discussion

Clothier: You criticized Warnock for not getting closer to public morality, or to what the man on the Clapham omnibus thinks. Of course that man is a fiction, he doesn't exist, just as the average man doesn't exist because he is made up of a very wide spectrum of different people with different opinions. What should the Warnock Committee have done, or what should we do now, to ascertain the common morality?

Hawthorn: You are quite right that there is no typical view but a collection of different views. It follows that there isn't a common morality in the strong sense or in the weakest sense, that is in the sense that there is agreement on what might be described as private morality.

I am certainly not suggesting that the Warnock Committee should have been guided by public opinion. The morality of ordinary people who don't have much time for reflection is determined in part by politics itself. In this kind of society, politics and all that may arise from it come in turn from technical advance. Certain things are made possible which were simply not envisaged earlier. Legislation and all the rest of it necessarily follow. If we had an alternative kind of society it would be very different but we are not talking about that. It doesn't follow that committees like Warnock should be guided exclusively by public opinion. My point was that that is one set of important opinions among others. It is a good deal more important than some but it is not overriding because none can be overriding.

Clothier: Opinion polls show that many people haven't thought about matters at all and don't have any opinion.

Hawthorn: Yes, such polls can also produce artificially clear and hard sets of opinions. They can predispose people towards saying 'yes' or 'no' because it is rather disgraceful to say 'don't know'. Pollsters now rephrase the 'don't know' part and say 'perhaps you haven't had time to think about it'. In the poll I described the proportion in that group was 25 per cent. In women in the reproductive age groups that proportion was much smaller; 25 per cent is an average of both sexes in the age group.

Williamson: I am not convinced that there is no consensus on common morality in this general area. These things change, and one of the problems in our discussions has been not examining the sense in which and the mechanisms by which they change. A Derby paediatrician was found not guilty of manslaughter when he clearly was, in the strictly technical, legal sense. A jury decided that that was not the way they saw the law. This is, in one sense, a moral or ethical decision derived by consensus. Do you really think there is no consensus on common morality?

Hawthorn: It depends what issue you are talking about, and what kind of morality. On this issue the short answer is no. Devlin believed that juries were the best tests of common opinion. But when he was writing juries had to be unanimous, and even now they have to come to a majority view. For this and other reasons (juries are, for instance, directed), I do not think that they can be taken to indicate very much. The polls suggest that the majority of people are perfectly happy for this treatment and the research associated with it to go ahead. But a clear minority, again about 25 per cent, are nervous. That nervousness may disappear, and it doesn't follow that one has to accept that as an incontrovertible, irreducible, unalterable, and practically obstructive fact. There will be debates on television, in the newspapers, and elsewhere. I take your point about change but there isn't a consensus. There is some artificiality in thinking of the typical man on the Clapham omnibus, or in having a committee that is going to produce a single view, but it doesn't follow that one has to take the minority opinion.

Williamson: There can be sufficient consensus to allow one to proceed.

Hawthorn: Yes, that's right.

Baird: The tenor of the discussion could perhaps be interpreted by saying that Warnock was deficient because not enough representative opinions were obtained. But they weren't set up to do that and when the Warnock Committee was set up there wasn't any information on those opinions. The National Opinion Poll you discussed was in July 1985 but I think our poll in Edinburgh (see Alder *et al.* 1986) was the first one that had done any kind of representative sampling. A women's magazine ran a poll about a year ago but they had two thousand replies from two million readers, which is 0.1 per cent of a selected population.

Reference

Alder, E.M., Baird, D.T., Lees, M.M., Lincoln, D., Loudon, N., and Templeton, A.A. (1986) Attitudes of women of reproductive age to *in vitro* fertilization and embryo research. *Journal of Biosocial Science*, submitted.

ELEVEN

Religions and the status of the embryo

J. W. Bowker

This paper considers the response of religions to the questions raised by embryo research. It makes the point that each religion is so diverse in itself that no uniform response in any one tradition can be expected. It then illustrates how in any case each religion creates a different anthropology, which in itself will produce different responses. Finally, the paper indicates how some of the traditions elaborate principles which they then apply to such unprecedented matters as the one under discussion at this meeting.

Since we have to cover a great deal of ground here let me say immediately that there is a practical wisdom in paying at least some attention to the attitudes of religious believers, if decisions have to be achieved which carry a consensus of opinion. That is so because the religious population of the world remains significant, and it does so even in this country, which happens to be about the most secular country in the most secular continent at the present time. Furthermore, the religious population even within this country, let alone in the world, is now extremely diverse, 'more Muslims than Methodists', as the saying goes.

It is entirely possible for the operators of systems (research units or research councils or whatever) to ignore religion as a 'vestigial remain' from the infancy of the human race. But that would be extremely unwise. It would ignore the fact that religions are extremely long-running and successful cultural packages, which have served well for the protection and enhancement of gene replication and for the nurture of successive generations.

The more deliberate, not to say aggressive, your ignoring of a religion is, the more likely you are to produce a defensive reaction of the kind we are familiar with in, say, Iran – and if you think Iran is a long way away and that it couldn't happen here, remember the strength and influence of the 'Moral Majority' in America. Maybe America is also a long way away; but if you act towards religions with a kind of pragmatic contempt, and without any attempts to understand why they are such successful and well-winnowed systems, you are likely to produce the phenomenon you most fear – highly conservative and defensive organizations which rightly perceive themselves to be under the attacks of indifference and contempt. I am not commenting on the truth or otherwise of what is being proposed in religious systems, only on the effect of regarding their concerns as negligible.

There is then a real wisdom in considering the attitudes of religions to major proposals that have to do, at least potentially, with human life. But that consideration is by no means easy to undertake. That is because no religion is a single entity; or, to put it another way, all religions are coalitions of immensely different ways of interpreting the fundamental resources available – and indeed, they may not agree on what *are* the fundamental resources and constraints. Thus there is no such thing as 'Christianity', only Catholic, Orthodox, Protestant interpretations of what it means to be Christian. There is no such thing as 'Judaism', only Orthodox, Liberal, Reform, and Progressive Jews. Hinduism makes a virtue of this evident necessity by calling itself not 'Hinduism', a word which is in any case a nineteenth century invention, but *Sanatana dharma* (*dharma* meaning roughly, 'discerning and doing what is appropriate for you in the particular circumstances in which you find yourself'); so that Hinduism is the map of *dharma*. So what the outsider calls Hinduism is a deliberate association of different routes to a goal, one of which may be appropriate for one individual, another for another.

The implication is obvious: in these religions there is not going to be a single, unanimous voice on any complex ethical issue. Consequently, anything I say on any of these traditions is disputable: neither I nor anyone else can 'speak for Hinduism' or 'speak for Buddhism'. The most we can hope for is to become aware of the way in which the issues occur as disputable within the traditions. But that gives us a most important point to hold on to. Since there is always an internal argument within religions on how to act, especially when unenvisaged or unprecedented circumstances occur, it is clearly in the interests of those who wish on their own grounds, whether moral *or* selfish, to engage in embryo research or genetic engineering, to participate in such internal arguments, at least to the extent of undertaking and reinforcing the arguments on their own side. That may well sound thoroughly cynical: it is not. It is simply realistic in observing that these unenvisaged or unprecedented issues are *open*: they are not yet resolved.

What do I mean by unenvisaged or unprecedented? Merely the obvious: that at the point where the fundamental resources of constraint and decision were laid down in these traditions, such issues as those of embryo research could not possibly be involved.

So all religions have to build bridges from the past to the present, and they do so with different procedures based on different identifications of what counts as fundamentally resourceful and of what its status is by way of authority. Thus there may be religions of revelation which establish what is in effect law, of which Orthodox Judaism, Islam, and Brahminical Hinduism are examples. Or there may be religions of revelation which establish principles, such as Christianity or types of Hinduism other than Brahminical. Or there may be religions of teaching which also establish principles, such as Buddhism.

None of these religions has anything specifically in its basic resource which deals with embryo research; so each has to use its own procedures for moving from the established past to the unenvisaged present. But clearly an issue they have in common is of whether embryo research is an engagement with a human life, or with human life, and, if so, whether such interaction or engagement is a fault or a virtue or neutral in relation to the principles regarding human life in each particular tradition. And that immediately complicates the scene much further, because there is no agreement between the different religions on what the nature of the human is; or, to put the matter more simply, each religion contains a totally different anthropology, a totally different reflection on what human nature is and, as we shall see, on when it begins.

Let me concentrate on one major issue of immediate and practical relevance: according to Western religions (with marginal exceptions in some expressions of Judaism), human life is constituted through the union of sperm and ovum and endowed with a particular form of life, or *nephesh*, or *nafs*, by God. In this context, it would not be inappropriate to translate this creative endowment by God as 'soul'. It may then be an issue when this created means of our relatedness to God and to each other appears as an emergent property or is bestowed as a necessary partner to the body; but in any case, it is not expected to persist in this 'vale of soul-making' for more than one appearance (with, as I say, minor exceptions in some expressions of Judaism, the *dibbuk* and the *gilgul*), and that appearance, according to the Psalmist, is not likely to be for longer than three score years and ten.

In the East it is entirely different. All Eastern religions believe that there are long sequences of continuity and that death is merely a means of transition to a new outcome – unless of course you can halt the process, or break outside it: and Eastern religions are there to indicate the procedures which make that emancipation, or release from the prison of rebirth, possible. Wittgenstein may have believed that death is not an event in life, but in the anthropology of Eastern religions it most certainly is. For unless and until you make that 'great escape', you may be reborn as many as eighty-four million times.

Of course, there is an issue between Hinduism and Buddhism about what is the 'you' or the 'I' which is being reborn: Hindus believe that the enduring, continuing, indestructible continuity in all things is Brahman – the unproduced producer of all that is. Brahman spills over into apparent forms – not least into theistic appearances which themselves, in divine exuberance, or *lila*, create other appearances beyond themselves. In humans, Brahman is present as *atman*; but as humans are diverted and become entangled in the material world, so *atman* becomes *jiva*, becomes the self unaware of its true nature. While it is entangled it is necessarily reborn over and over again in the forms to which it is most attached: thus the poor man who longs for the riches of a Getty or a Kennedy will be reborn in the form to which he is attached, with all the wealth he desired – and will, of course, discover its ultimate emptiness.

The 'skill-in-means' of Hinduism (though that is in fact a Buddhist phrase) is to work back to such a point that the *jiva* realizes its proper identity as *atman*, and as *atman* its true nature as Brahman, as what it is – not only *what* there is, but also *why* it is at all. Hence we get the sequence shown in the diagram (Fig. 11.1).

Brahman underlies all appearance, and becomes manifest in those forms of appearance which are called 'gods'. In divine exuberance (*lila*) universes are formed, and humans appear. Brahman underlies them as *atman*, but in entanglement the self as *jiva* is continuously reborn, in a cycle of rebirth. But when *jiva* realizes that its true nature is *atman*, and that *atman* is Brahman, it can return (*moksha*) to its true identity. So Hinduism as *Sanatana dharma* is the enduring means of showing you how to act for the best, how to act appropriately, how to act in this particular birth, to move yourself closer to *moksha*, to release. In any birth you may be at one of many levels, depending on *karma* – on the consequences running on from your previous births – so that

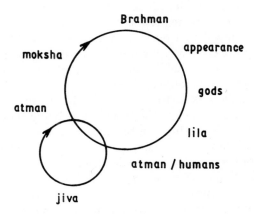

Figure 11.1

karma itself has determined the condition in which you have been born: hence the caste system simply formalizes *dharma*. But in general Hinduism recognizes that there are different *purusartha* – goals in life: *abhyudaya*, appropriate goals in relation to the world and this life; and *nihsreyasa*, spiritual goals which may increasingly disregard the former.

In general an individual is likely (and according to the Manusmriti is obliged) to move through the four *asramas*, or stages of life: student; householder; the one who withdraws from full engagement in life; and the complete renouncer or total ascetic; and what is appropriate for each of those stages will clearly vary.

So, in this context, abortion might be legitimate to save the life of the mother, so that she can sustain her own dharmic role in relation to the existing family, even if that is, to that point, restricted to her husband.

Equally, there is no intrinsic objection to contraception: 'Now the woman whom one desires [with the thought] "may she not conceive", after inserting the penis in her, joining mouth to mouth, he should inhale, then exhale, and say, "with power, with semen, I reclaim the semen from you". Thus, she comes to be without seed' [Brhadaranyaka Up. 6.iv.10].

However, those considerations do not create a general licence: in general, Hindu social ethics rest on *lokasamgraha*, care of the *loka*, or world, as the Gita puts it: 'it was by works that Janaka and others attained to perfection. You should do works also with a view to the maintaining of the world' [iii.20].

In that more general context, it is a deep offence, with karmic consequence, to kill any sentient being; and that includes abortion, even when it is accepted as the lesser evil. Certainly killing an embryo, *bhruna hatya*, comes within this consideration; and because of the sense of *atman/jiva* sequentially and consequentially uniting with a new life (a zygote) *ab initio*, discussions of hominization or ensoulment at a later date are not relevant to a Hindu anthropology. The overriding control is *ahimsa*, non-violence; and in virtually all Hindu systems *ahimsa* is not relative: its scope is universal; and Gandhi simply applied it in one particular domain.

To take just one example: the system of Patanjali lists the

astanga yoga, the eightfold means of Yoga. The first of these is restraint, *yama*. What components constitute *yama*? The first is *ahimsa*, which is attitude as well as action – it is non-hatred (*vairatyaga*) as well as non-violence.

The commentary on this makes it clear that the scope of *ahimsa* is universal – as Cromwell Crawford (1982, p. 99) summarizes the point: 'Its scope is universal. It is "not limited" by life-state, space, time and circumstance' [ii.30]. That is to say, *ahimsa* cannot be relativized by a series of 'ifs', 'ands', and 'buts'.

Thus the fisherman cannot say, 'Well, I won't injure anything except for fish'; and a soldier cannot say, 'I won't injure anything except in battle'. 'Universal is that which pervades all conditions of life, everywhere, always, and is nowhere out of place. They are called the great vow.' [*Yoga Bhasya* ii.31.]

But notice 'the great vow': this is a willed movement into an absolute condition. As it stands, without that formal transition, it conflicts with *dharma*, particularly with the precise issue of *dharma* which evoked the Bhagavad Gita – the Song of the Lord Krishna, which is part of the Ramayana, and which is for many Hindus their most revered scripture. The *Gita* is evoked by a circumstance where a warrior, Arjuna, turns away from battle, because his own kinsmen are on the other side. But Krishna tells him that it is his *dharma*, his appropriate way of acting as a warrior, to engage in the battle; and then he reinforces that argument by appealing to the implications of Hindu anthropology: if it is Brahman, the unproduced producer of all that is, which is in all appearance as its underlying and enduring reality, then it is not possible to *kill* the essential reality of anything. Yes, indeed, you may kill the outward appearance, the manifest form of the body, but you cannot kill *it*. So we arrive at the famous passage in the Gita, that there is neither killer nor killed, neither slayer nor slain.

In that context, the *dharma* of the doctor is to help and to heal, and to do such things as will enhance that probability, as, for example, knowing the conjunction of stars and knowing the auspicious time to operate; but also, for another example, undertaking necessary research.

So we see that a case can be made for embryo research which accepts, as with abortion, that it is a grievous offence, but which subserves the *dharma* of the doctor. It is simply that the doctor is far from *moksha*, release, and from yet being able to undertake the great vow. But by acting dharmically *as* a doctor, he will of course move closer, through rebirth, to the ideal of *ahimsa*.

Ahimsa, non-violence, is even more strongly emphasized in two protest movements against Hinduism, the Jains and the Buddhists. In the Hindu Upanishads, there is only one reference to *ahimsa*, in a passage which remythologizes sacrifice and says that the *daksina*, or gift for the priests, can be performed, not only by the sacrificial gifts, but equally by the spiritual donation of 'austerity, almsgiving, uprightness, *ahimsa*, and truthfulness' [Chandogya Up. 3.17.4]. But in Buddhism, non-violence has worked its way even into the Five Precepts, the five basic promises which a Buddhist makes to himself every day.

But the Buddhist makes that promise in relation to a divergent anthropology. Buddhists believe that there is continuity from life to life to life, through as many reappearances as the Hindus believe that there are rebirths; but for the Buddhist, nothing is being reborn. In other words, there is no self, or *atman*, moving on through the long sequences of birth. For the Buddhist, there is only the flow of available energy aggregating into forms of appearance, like shoes and ships and sealing wax and cabbages and kings. But the flow of aggregation is consequential: it is as much governed by *karma* as it is for Hindus. So each moment gives rise to the next, not because there is a self or soul giving continuity to the process, but because the process is governed by regularities as immutable as the force of attraction between masses which we refer to as gravity.

Here at least, one would think, embryo research should be unproblematic, because there is no interacting with an inviolable soul, but only with an aggregation of particular availabilities, whose *dhamma* (since Buddhists have a comparable concept to *dharma*) might be to be experimented on.

But in fact it is not as simple as that, because although Buddhists maintain *anatta*, no-soul, they also maintain that the five *khandhas*, the five aggregates which constitute human being, appear in the sort of complexity which demands respect and *ahimsa*, non-violence.

Furthermore, that respect must apply to the earliest moment, because although there is no 'self' going on from one life to another, there is real continuity of consequence which jumps on from the moment of death to the moments of new aggregation or appearance: the thread is continuous, although it is below the level of surface self-aware consciousness. The karmic consequence is carried across to a new appearance – traditionally by the remythologized but nevertheless still mythical figure of the *gandhabba*. What that means is a belief that the process of continuity is co-terminous with conception, and that such considerations as those of twinning or recombination will be interpreted as themselves karmically caused. This is how a modern Western interpreter of Buddhism, the Mahathera Nyanatiloka, summarized the point (see Collins 1982, p. 213):

> According to Buddhism, there are three factors necessary for the rebirth of a human being, that is, for the formation of the embryo in the mother's womb. They are: the female ovum, the male sperm, and the *karma*-energy, *kamma-vega*, which in the *Suttas* is metaphorically called the *gandhabba*, i.e. 'ghost'. This *karma*-energy is sent forth by a dying individual at the moment of his death. Father and mother only provide the necessary physical material for the formation of the embryonic body. With regard to the characteristic features, the tendencies and faculties lying latent in the embryo, the Buddha's teaching may be explained in the following way: the dying individual with his whole being convulsively clinging to life, at the very moment of his death, sends forth *karmic* energies which, like a flash of lightning, hit at a new mother's womb ready for conception. Thus, through the impinging of the *karma*-energies on the ovum and the sperm, there arises, just as a precipitate, the so-called primary cell.

It is impossible in Buddhism to identify a space before the embryo, in the Buddhist sense, becomes human, because the thread is continuous.

The absolute seriousness of this can be seen in the resurgence of the *mizugo* prayer in Japan, in response to the increase in abortions: the *mizugo* is the aggregation constituting human appearance in the stages before birth, of which, in Buddhist analysis, there are five, beginning with the very moment of conception. The *mizugo* prayer and ritual does for the pre-birth dead what one would do for any of the family dead after birth.

Thus Domyo Miura comments (see Miura 1983, p. 14, p. 26f):

> Buddhism takes the stand that the right to life for all beings must be respected. For example, even before a child actually comes into the world, Buddhists regard it as a life from the very instant when consciousness is born. . . .[1] When life is produced in the womb at conception, this is termed 'maku no toki', . . . A *mizugo's* existence begins at that stage produced by conception, which in modern parlance means that life is seen to start from the instant the sperm joins with the egg.

Domyo Miura is himself the leader of the Enmanin Temple, near Kyoto in Japan, part of whose purpose is to enable the *mizugo* prayer to pass the unborn on to its next destiny, assisted as it would be if it had died after birth. There is no candidate here for delayed hominization, as there has been in the West, with various thresholds proposed, ranging from birth itself, back through viability and the formation of the cerebral cortex, to the point at which it is settled whether there will be one or two or more distinct human individuals.

In contrast, some Western religions *have* identified stages, especially in relation to abortion. In Islam, a consensus was reached that a foetus becomes a person when it receives its soul from God, which was generally agreed to be at the end of the fourth month.

The majority of the jurists in the four main Muslim schools of law (Hanifite, Hanbalite, Malikite, and Shafiite) agree that there can be no abortion after this unless it is reliably established that to continue the pregnancy would endanger the life of the mother.

But they failed to reach any consensus on abortion *before* that time – in contrast to the way in which they did agree that there are circumstances in which, for example, contraception is legitimate; and for those who do allow abortion before that time, abortion is accepted with contraception as a form of birth control.

Thus, the Zaydis, at an extreme, maintained that the unformed

---

[1] Consciousness, here, does not depend on the development of the cerebral cortex – a candidate for some, in the Western debate, for the moment of hominization and the acquisition of rights. What is referred to here is the *bhavanga* substrate of identity, as in deep sleep, when active consciousness is not evident.

(i.e. unensouled) foetus is in the same condition as semen, i.e. without human life. Consequently, abortion is possible un-conditionally – it is not necessary to give a sufficient reason for it.

The Hanifites say that it is possible only with sufficient reason, that, for example, the pregnant mother is still breast-feeding another infant.

The Malikites agree that it is not a human being, but they anticipate the view of Pope Paul VI (1973, p. 4ff), that it is *personne en devenir*: consequently, it should never be disturbed or interfered with, except in the most exceptional circumstances.

So this might seem to leave open the possibility of 'unsettled embryo' research, much more obviously than is the case in Eastern religions. The Quran itself envisages stages of growth:

> O men, if you are in doubt about the resurrection, surely we created you out of dust, then out of sperm, then out of a small clot, then out of a morsel of flesh, formed and unformed, in order that we may demonstrate to you; and we cause what we will to rest in the wombs for an appointed term, then do we bring you out as infants, then that you may reach your full strength; and some of you are called to die, and some are kept back to the most abject life. [xxii.5.]
>
> He created you from a single *nafs*, then he created from it a partner. . . . He makes you in the wombs of your mothers in stage [*halqan*] after stage in three darknesses [*fi zulumathin thalathin*]: that is God your Lord; to him is all authority. [xxxix.6/8.]
>
> We created man from a lump of clay, then we placed him as a sperm in a place of rest, secure; then we made the sperm into a clot, then we made the clot into a form, then we made the form into bones and clothed the bones with flesh. Then we developed it as another creature. [xxiii.12ff.]

So perhaps at an early stage, there might be a case for experiment on the equivalent of lifeless tissue. However, for Islam this suggestion runs into the objection of an immensely strong doctrine of creation: to create life in order to end it is to rival the actions which belong only to God. The drawing of pictures of living people or animals is itself prohibited in Islam on exactly these grounds, let alone the actual evocation of life outside the context of intended birth. In any case, even where abortion is concerned, it is an offence at *any* stage for most Muslims (not all,

as we have seen), but in differing degrees. So alGhazali summarizes the consensus (in alQaradawi 1981, p. 202):

> Contraception is not like abortion. Abortion is a crime against an
> existing being. Now, existence has stages. The first stages of existence
> are the setting of the semen in the womb and its mixing with the
> secretions of the woman. It is then ready to receive life. Disturbing it
> is a crime. When it develops further and becomes as a lump, aborting
> it is a greater crime. When it acquires a soul and its creation is
> completed, the crime becomes more grievous. The crime reaches a
> maximum seriousness, when it is committed after it is separated alive
> (from the mother).

Islam places a high value on *ilm*, knowledge, and led the first
renaissance of Greek science and the renewal of medicine as a
result, with such figures as arRhazi dominating the Western
world long after his death. But *ilm* has boundaries, derived from
the sense of God as sole creator, which cannot be transcended, and
which many Muslims certainly think *would* be transcended by
producing embryos not for birth but for research.

But it is not a unanimous voice: others hold that this is human
tissue but not human life, as we have seen in connection with
abortion.

On abortion, Jews also make a distinction of periods, between
early and late, though there is some dispute about the boundary;
usually it is forty days (by rabbinic calculation), certainly never
more than three months. In *all* periods, as Klein puts it, 'the law is
clear and explicit: the mother's life must be saved even at the cost
of the life of the foetus of the unborn child, at any stage of the
pregnancy as long as the child is in the womb. In the early period
therapeutic abortion is allowed on the grounds *'ubbar yerek 'immo
hu*, that the foetus is a limb of the mother, or in Roman law *pars
viscerum matris'* (Klein 1979, p. 416). In other words, the
operation is really on part of the mother, not on another human
being. Since there is a consensus that mental health is on a par
with physical health, abortions may be permitted in the early
period for a wide range of reasons, including the fear of bearing a
deformed child as a result of German measles or drugs such as
thalidomide.

All this occurs within the Orthodox domain. Might it then lead to an equivalent of the Zaydi position, that experimentation on embryos is equally permissible? Staying within the Orthodox domain, the answer is clearly not, and many non-Orthodox Jews would agree, not least because of memories recalled by the present Chief Rabbi: 'One need only recall the horrors of the Nazi practices "in the services of medicine" to realise the diabolical excesses to which the sacrifice of human rights for medical research can lead' (Jakobovitz 1975, p. 291).

Does the embryo have human rights? Well, clearly, as we have just seen, that is not a particularly intelligible question in Judaism. Such rights as it has are related to the mother, not to issues of when it is ensouled, or when it is ready to partake in the *'olam haBa*, the world to come.

But it is not negligible either: it is related to *life, ab initio*. And since all human life is equally valuable and inviolable, including that of 'criminals, prisoners, and defectives', to quote the usual list, and one life cannot be sacrificed to save another or even any number of others, there is certainly strong Jewish opinion that to produce embryos for experimentation is to produce an unacceptable divovce fvom the locus of decision in relation to the mother.

But it is not a unanimous voice. Since there is that very distinction, work to combat such genetic diseases as Tay-Sachs disease (which is markedly present in the Jewish community) is held to be justified.

We have seen, therefore, that the attitudes in different religions are extremely diverse and by no means uniform in each tradition. The same is true of Christianity, which is not dealt with in this paper, because the participants in this meeting who are speaking out of the Christian tradition make it clear how great the differences between them are. By no means do all people in all religions regard pre-embryo research as precluded on the grounds that a person with rights is initiated from the point of conception. Nevertheless, if one is hoping for some reasonable consensus in society, it is all the more important not to evade the hardest case (on the grounds that it is not unanimously held) but take, as Hardy put it, 'a full look at the worst'.

In this respect, there is no doubt that many people in religious traditions do believe there is an important degree of novelty at the formation of the zygote, or at least, to add Ramsey's qualifier, 'from the time at or after which it is settled whether there will be one or two or more distinct human individuals' – though, as we have just seen, Eastern religions would not necessarily accept that qualification, and some moral theologians in the West (e.g. R.A. McCormick) would say that while the qualifier is disputed, 'benefit of the doubt should ordinarily be given to the foetus'. But let us accept the hardest feasible case, of the *personne en devenir*, not in the germ-line but in the zygote.

What then needs to be explored in all religions, and indeed outside them, is what decisions can legitimately and morally be made on their behalf, since they clearly have no utterance of their own. *Abstract* considerations of human rights are not well founded in that case; for what we are considering here are the 'rights of the voiceless', to use the technical phrase. Through long centuries of moral reflection, we have found it puzzling, but not impossible, to make decisions on behalf of the voiceless at the other end of life. We do, as a matter of fact, make decisions on behalf of the incompetent when they are very old and when they are approaching death. We do, incidentally, make decisions on behalf of the (technically) incompetent in the case of children. What informs such decisions? Clearly one component in such decisions is a resounding answer to the question (which is at least as old as Socrates) whether death is as great an evil as we suppose – an emphatic answer, No, it is not the greatest evil, necessarily, that we can suppose.

The implication of that is that while human life is a basic good and is the foundation for the enjoyment of other goods and rights, it does not follow that life *cannot* be taken when doing so is the lesser of two evils, all things considered as far as they can be; or, which is more characteristic of religions, if it is the greater of two goods. That is readily translatable into the earlier discussion of *dharma*. It is from that kind of consideration that soldiers can be asked, and morally expected (at least in some circumstances), to fight to kill; and that justification of taking life occurs in Buddhism, just as it does in other religions.

What is then usually argued is that, to qualify as the lesser of two evils, a human life or its moral equivalent must be at issue. What is meant by 'moral equivalent'? Is there some good or value that is equivalent to life itself?

Obviously that evaluation of equivalence is itself difficult: but in the case of the just war, for example, the comparison is that, if human beings may go to war and take human life to defend their freedom (i.e. political autonomy, freedom to dispense of themselves by some kind of agreed consensus), then that freedom is being compared with human life.

So it is at the other end of life, in relation to death, that we already have some consideration of the lesser of two evils, and the greater of two goods, and we have much more established discussion in the exploration of proxy consent for termination of life – and also of proxy consent to therapy for a child's good; and what is traditionally considered here is what the child would choose on the basis of what he or she should (ought to) choose, given that she or he ought to choose the good of life as long as this life remains, all things considered, a human good.

What about therapy for others? If we ask young people to die in a just war, might we ask embryos to die in a just (i.e. justifiable) war against a specific defect, e.g. a genetic defect, of the kind mentioned frequently in this symposium?

In that case the Helsinki declaration would be being affirmed on behalf of the voiceless. Some religions (e.g. that particular voice of Judaism which I have already quoted) would necessarily object. But for others (and I think, when it is tied to the religious notion of sacrifice, that it might be a majority), this is acceptable. *Of course*, it imposes limits – the experiment must be necessary and proportionate to the goals; it could not produce but only accept embryos; it should not usually promote harm in order simply to study its own effect; and so on. But in general this approach does not rule out such actions on the ground that no infant would or could assent. Rather, it emphasizes that *because* they are human, but not yet able to speak for themselves, we have to make the best human judgement that we can suppose they would make when competent.

The formula which Stephen Toulmin proposed was, 'What may it be presumed that the foetus *could not reasonably object to*, if it were capable . . . ?' (Toulmin 1975, pp. 31–5).

I prefer to put it more positively – and I know to some it sounds more facetiously – when I ask whether it makes moral sense to say, 'Greater love hath no pre-embryo than this, that it lay down its life that cannot come to term for the more abundant life of others' – life on the other side of the healing of infertility, genetic defects, and the like.

Not all religions accept that principle of sacrifice. But most do, somewhere: and Christianity, I believe, can do so with a good conscience.

This means, paradoxically, that discussions of religious reflections on the treatment of the origin of life in the embryo need to consider first the religious evaluation of death – not of life in isolation from the whole process of evolution, in which human life is possible only as a consequence of death.

References

Collins, S. (1982) *Selfless Persons*. Cambridge University Press

Crawford, S.C. (1982) *The Evolution of Hindu Ethical Ideals*, 2nd edn. Hawaii University Press, Honolulu

Diamond, J.J. (1974) Pro-life amendments and due process. *America*, pp. 27–9

Jakobovitz, I. (1975) *Jewish Medical Ethics*, 2nd edn. New York: Bloch

Klein, I. (1979) *A Guide to Jewish Practice*. New York: Jewish Theological Seminary

Miura, D. (1983) *The Forgotten Child*. Henley: Aidan Ellis

Pope Paul VI (1973) Pourquoi l'église ne peut accepter l'avortement. *Documentation Catholique* LXX

alQaradawi, Y. (1981) *The Lawful and the Prohibited in Islam*. Indianapolis: American Trust Publications

Toulmin, S. (1975) Exploring the moderate consensus. *Hastings Center Report* 5: 31–35

Discussion

Clothier: Because reputable people have shown me that it happens I can believe that at the fourteenth day an important change comes over the cluster of cells we are discussing. I can define 'believing' in a particular way there. If I were to say that I believe I may live for ever I would have to redefine the word believe. Does the theory of human existence that you described help us to solve the practical question of the point at which the embryo becomes entitled to a special regard or the point at which we owe it the duty of a special regard? Does Hinduism or any other religion offer a choice of points?

Bowker: Not 'theory' but 'theories': since each religion maintains a different anthropology (i.e. a different account of human nature), each religion will identify differently the moment when *human* life (and therefore the attribution of such rights and obligations as that particular tradition also maintains) begins. In that sense, the religions do not help but hinder, because they complicate the quest for consensus in a society such as ours, which is religiously pluralistic in such an obvious way. The additional question which you raise is whether, if there was an abortion for the sake of the mother in the seventh month, you could then experiment on the aborted foetus. Those who agree with the position I put forward at the end of my paper would say you could.

Clothier: The aborted foetus is dead but the embryo is alive and capable of further development.

Bowker: People with religious convictions would not try to abort it alive, but if it happened that the foetus was alive when it was aborted I think some could say that you could experiment on it if there was no possibility of bringing it to term. Whatever is done would always be in the context of ritual attitudes of respect. The Methodist church has just questioned whether there should be a prayer for the aborted foetus. Japanese religion has the *mizugo* prayer in relation to the aborted foetus, with ritualized actions of respect and recognition that this is human continuity, apparent in human form.

Dunstan: In what sense are you using the words embryo and foetus in your paper, Professor Bowker?

Bowker: It will be different in different religions. The diversity of language is a way of drawing attention to the diversity of significant dates in different religions. That is going to be confusing.

McLaren: The term foetus is normally used from about eight weeks after ovulation, that is ten weeks after the last menstrual period. Embryo applies to the entity that begins to develop about sixteen days after ovulation, and pre-embryo applies before that, for the totality of cells that arise from the fertilized egg.

Clothier: What happens at eight weeks to change the name?

Baird: It looks like a wee baby.

Edwards: Professor Bowker pointed out that some religions would balance the respective benefits of making a decision on embryo research and whether the embryo should be sacrificed for this purpose. This is not alien to our thought either. There has been a lot of debate, especially among scientists, that any damage done to the embryo could be balanced by a greater good for the adult or young person who has an illness or a genetic defect. Perhaps we reach similar conclusions by a different route.

Maddox: The practical problem is how one defines regulatory regimes in a multiracial and multireligious society like ours where people will inevitably have very different estimates of the importance of the embryo. At one end of the spectrum one has people like me who would say that the moral status of the embryo is no different from that of animals that are bred to be eaten, which is not to say they have no right to respect. At the other extreme there are people who would altogether forbid embryo research. The question then is, to what extent will people at this second extreme tolerate work by others closer to the other extreme? Do the religions you talked about admit of tolerance of what happens in the society in which they belong?

Bowker: The further east you go the more tolerant they are, in your sense. The clearest examples are the Jains. They have formally worked it out that as you are reborn so many times you have to accept that other people are at different stages in the long process. Therefore Jains, for example, will accept that others can kill animals or can be cobblers who use leather. In Eastern religions, it is built into the anthropology that you accept that others will eventually reach your stage of enlightenment, or that you will probably start again where they are now. The difficulty for Christianity is how to learn to live with competing interpretations. The articulation of tolerance in Christianity is always there but in practice it is a great problem. On what terms does Christianity live with others who disagree as profoundly as they do on this question?

Clothier: They didn't tolerate each other very well in the partition of India.

Bowker: Gandhi was killed by two orthodox Hindus because they thought this was against the *dharma* of a ruler looking after the resources of a country. He contradicted the *dharma*. The *dharma* may make it appropriate to kill.

Hull: In this discussion we are talking about sacrifice and harm or hurt. To me sensibility is the key question. Is the view of the foetus as a sentient being the traditional view in Hinduism? Has there been recent discussion of what we now call the early embryo and its sentience?

Bowker: There has certainly been a lot of discussion. There is a sort of *dharma* towards plant life, though this is more likely to be in Buddhism. Ultimately when you are going to the fourth stage of Hindu life, of total withdrawal, you start to die, say thirty to forty years before the event. You gradually leave behind all the pain that you might cause to even the plant life. In the end nobody is feeding you, you are not feeding yourself, and you just drift away. It is a form of long-term suicide. The discussion in Hinduism always comes back to the hardest case. You have to act towards this tissue, or this pre-embryo, as towards the *Brahman* underlying it. But the *dharma* of the doctor or the researcher or the farmer cutting corn is that they must do it thoroughly and well, or they will not proceed toward release from the cycle of rebirth. If researchers held back from some procedure which might lead to a cure of a genetic defect, they would be failing in their *dharma*. Sacrifice is thus a good term. It is not just life giving way to life, but life giving way so that other life can come into existence. This is the key insight. Hindus believe that the whole universe is a great sacrifice, devourer, devouring, and devoured. A doctor is participating, if you like, in the great sacrifice of the universe and is enabling life through the process of death.

Hull: When we are concerned about the individual who is being sacrificed it seems to me we can only apply the term to a being that is sentient. If that being is not sentient, then we don't have to talk about evil or good, and we do not need to apply the term sacrifice in any way.

Bowker: In terms of the equivalent of proxy consent and recognizing what you are doing with this pre-embryo or embryo, it is built in that this sequence is on the human line. In other words, Hindus may be disagreeing with you, because they want to say let us treat it as quasi-human, or indeed as human, and *still* say this is right. It is really taking the hardest possible case, without stepping around it and saying that this is pre-human or something like that. It is *Brahman* manifesting itself in appearance, and we are going to treat it as human and make these decisions on its behalf, according to its own *dharma*.

Hull: What I am trying to avoid is the need to defend a position which I don't think we have to defend.

Braude: There are some concepts prompted by the development of fertilization *in vitro* that religions have not had to deal with before. For instance, 'life' and 'alive' are often dealt with in a confusing manner. If we take a fertilized egg and keep it in culture, rather than returning it to a uterus, we can grow sheets of cells from it (cell lines) and keep these growing in culture indefinitely. Although some may like to believe that the starting material, a fertilized egg, is 'life', it is clear that no 'life' has or can now derive from it, despite the fact that the cells are still alive.

Bowker: Religions do deal with those concepts now, maybe inadequately. Many Indian and Japanese doctors just get on with their work without paying attention to this kind of thinking. Some of them will probably agree with your point of view that linking the traditional religious views to this kind of question is misleading. My view is that it is probably a mistake to ignore the sensitivities of religious traditions, because it is not automatic that societies will sustain scientific enterprise, no matter how many technological goods come from it. The recovery of Greek science and medicine in Islam stopped very abruptly in the Ottoman empire. Equally to the point, these religions do not accept that there is no empirical foundation for their views. In the eastern religions there are three components for conception: the egg, the seed, and the karmic consequence. They think they have empirical evidence for it. The karmic onflow will connect up with what has been conceived and brought into being. Consequently, from the outset it is a human individual, but, as I have said, that does not rule out some action in relation to it, in the context of *dharma* and sacrifice.

TWELVE

Types of moral argument against embryo research

B. Williams

Almost all moral objections to embryo research depend on one version or another of a *slippery slope* argument. There is one absolutist consideration which may be thought to decide the question independently of that argument, to the effect that the early embryo simply is a human being. But any plausible use of that consideration itself relies on the slippery slope argument. This argument may use either of two ideas (or both): that to distinguish between the two cases is not *reasonable* or that it will not be *effective*. The argument turns out to be very largely an empirical, consequentialist argument, and its application to early embryo research to rest on doubtful assumptions.

I shall not try to consider every form of moral argument that has been brought to bear on these questions. I shall concentrate for the most part on a matter that is important to very many of them, the use of 'slippery slope' considerations.

I should like to start by making one or two points about the Warnock Report (see Warnock 1985). It has been held against the report that it lacks a theoretical base. This criticism seems to me to be both ambiguous and for the most part misplaced. It may mean that the report contains no arguments: that is simply untrue. It may mean that the Committee had no reflective understanding of what they were doing: that seems to me, also, untrue. What is true is that they do not base their conclusions on some ethical theory, such as utilitarianism. That is true, but seems to me to be sensible. Some utilitarian considerations – that is to say, consequentialist considerations concerned with welfare – must play a role in any sensible discussion of these matters, and I shall be concerned with them in talking about the slippery slope. But to try to derive a knock-down answer to these problems by applying the simple utilitarian theory is just as arbitrary as to rely on unexamined prejudices – it may merely be simpler. Again, the invocation of a theory of rights is likely to lead to indeterminate results in a question of this kind; we need some more reflection on what people feel about these matters before we can confidently begin to appeal to such notions.

I therefore do not see much wrong with what I take to be basically Warnock's method, which is to think as hard as possible about the implications of deeply held ethical views. That approach does raise two very important questions. First, what is it for ethical or moral attitudes to be 'deeply held'? It is certainly not the same thing as their being emphatically expressed, as often seems to be supposed. Reflection is needed to discover how deeply enmeshed certain outlooks or attitudes are in our understanding of ourselves, of human life, and of society. There are some points at which Warnock's argument seems to me, at least, not to have taken this question far enough; the views on surrogacy, in particular, seem to have been added to the rest of the argument on principles that are respectable rather than profound.

The second question that is raised by such a method is: *whose* ethical views are under examination? Or, since they are certainly *ours*, who is meant by 'we'? Here one has to remember that what Warnock's discussion was directed at was legislation; and presumably our discussions here, even if participants may take different views about the desirability of legislation, are fundamentally concerned with questions of regulation. Thus each of us has to consider, not just what he or she feels about this matter, but what it is reasonable to put into legislation for a community such as ours. [The point that our community is very various and pluralistic, particularly from the point of view of religion, was made in the discussion, notably by John Maddox.]

Warnock starts from a moral assumption that the Committee takes us to share: 'Every one agrees that it is completely unacceptable to make use of a child or an adult as the subject of research procedure which may cause harm or death' [para. 11.12]. I take it that everyone taking part in this discussion shares that assumption, as I do. Some people no doubt do not share that assumption: there are some philosophers who do not, or say that they do not. I share the assumption, and I am glad to say that since it is shared (at present) by a large majority of the community, it is going to be the starting point of any acceptable legislation. Granted this assumption, the question of embryo experiment, like the questions raised by abortion, immediately raises the matter of the slippery slope. Is there any line that it can be sensible or appropriate to draw between experiment on a neonate, which is rejected, and experiment on an early embryo? What would be involved in drawing such a line?

There are one or two points to be made about slippery slope arguments in general, a question I have discussed elsewhere (Williams 1986). All slippery slope arguments take the form of claiming that if a certain practice or act is allowed, we shall end up with an unacceptable result, because there is a series of cases between the original case and the unacceptable outcome, and none of them can be distinguished from its neighbours. So if A is allowed, there will be no way of distinguishing B from it, or distinguishing C from B, and so on, until an unacceptable result is reached. Within this general formula, there are two significant distinctions to be made. We should distinguish two different kinds of 'unacceptable result' to which slippery slope arguments may appeal. In some cases, what is appealed to is a *horrible* result: the slope is thought to lead to some practice which in itself is horrible, morally unacceptable, etc. This is the case with such arguments when applied to embryo experiment and abortion, the horrible result being, of course, the state of affairs in which neonates are experimented on or killed. But in other sorts of case, the slippery slope argument appeals rather to what may be called an *arbitrary* result. In such cases, the objection is not that the slope necessarily arrives at some particular hideous class of practices; the objection is rather that once one has crossed the first line, there is simply no way of drawing any line at all.

An example of this would be a situation in which, as things are, a certain social benefit is allowed only to legally married couples. It is proposed that the benefit be extended to couples who are not legally married; some people objected to this that they did not mind the mere idea of such benefit being given to people who are not married, but once the clear rule requiring legal marriage had been abandoned, there simply was no satisfactory criterion at all by which it could be determined which couples might have the benefit and which not. The objection in this case would be to the arbitrariness of the outcome, not to its intrinsic horribleness.

Another distinction that needs to be made about such arguments concerns what is meant by the claim that a case 'cannot be distinguished' from its neighbours. It is important to be clear whether this means, in a given example, that two cases cannot be *reasonably* distinguished, or that they cannot *effectively* be distinguished. It is one thing to ask whether the difference between two cases is reasonably related to the subject matter in hand, based on a consideration of principle, etc.; and it is another thing to ask whether a distinction will actually stick, whether in psychological or social terms a line will be held between one kind of case and the next. This is illustrated by the case of regimes to regulate eating or smoking. The difference between no cigarettes or chocolates a day, and one cigarette or chocolate a day, is smaller, in terms of what those items do to the body, than the distinction between one cigarette or chocolate a day, and thirty. Indeed, in terms of harm done, one cigarette or chocolate a day may be insignificant, but making a rule demanding no cigarettes rather than one may be the only psychologically effective step, just because one a day leads to thirty a day, while none a day does not.

When we are concerned with social practices and public rules, it is always important to consider what forces may be at work to extend some practice to new kinds of case, and to move us further down the slippery slope. In the addiction case, pressure to consume more cigarettes or chocolates is exercised by well-known psychological forces; in social cases, one has to have a realistic picture of the forces that will be at work. Will there be an interest operating to extend the practice? In some cases, there evidently is – this is likely to be so in the case of claiming social benefits, for instance. In other cases, it may be a fantasy that there is continuous latent pressure to move further down the slippery slope; a moralistic model of addiction may be at work. In this connection, I think that it is important that the public is suspicious of motivations that obtain in the medical profession; an image of medical workers fanatically devoted to experiment may play a suspect role in the argument.

Slightly different from the question whether there is constant pressure of the addictive kind to move down the slope, there is the matter of habituation, by which the last case that was accepted simply seems less extreme after it has been accepted than it did before. Here a cognitive process is in question, and another example of it, in a different connection, is that which has been invoked by the American philosopher Nelson Goodman to explain the fact that certain art experts were prepared at one time to accept as genuine paintings by Vermeer a series of increasingly crude and unconvincing forgeries by Van Meegeren. Goodman's idea is that each new forgery was compared to a reference class of supposed Vermeers which included the previous forgeries, and it was only when Van Meegeren was exposed, and each forgery was compared to a reference class that excluded the others, that the crudity of the later ones became apparent. A rather similar process may be invoked to explain how social practice might possibly move down a slope. The possibility may be presented, in some cases, in unduly moralistic terms, but it is a possible process, and should be taken into account in any serious calculation of the effects of introducing social practices that raise this kind of question.

Just as we have to distinguish between the claims that a distinction is intrinsically reasonable, and that it is effective, so we also have to distinguish between a distinction's being unreasonable, in terms of the original subject matter, and its being ineffective. When the slippery slope is invoked we need to consider not merely what distinctions of principle can be drawn, but what distinctions are likely to have, or fail to have, a social effect. It is because we can make these distinctions, that the possibility of a slippery slope does not necessarily prove that we should never start; even when there is a real social possibility of sliding down a slope, that does not necessarily show that the first step should not be taken. There is an alternative, which is to *draw a line*, and that is the method that Warnock recommended with regard to embryo experiment. The Warnock Report is extremely clear that its recommended time limit of fourteen days for such experiment is indeed a regulatory line; though it bears a rough relation to a salient developmental feature, it is not intended to be an approximation to some characteristic which might be thought in itself relevant to the issue of experiment, such as sentience.

Is drawing a line in this way reasonable? Can it be effective? The answer to both these questions seems to me to be 'yes, sometimes', and, as that unexciting reply suggests, there is not a great deal to be brought to deciding them beyond good sense and relevant information. It may be said that a line of this kind cannot possibly be reasonable since it has to be drawn between two adjacent cases in the range, that is to say, between two cases that are not different enough to distinguish. The answer is that they are indeed not different enough to distinguish if that means that their characteristics, unsupported by anything else, would have led one to draw a line there. But though the line is not, in this sense, uniquely reasonable, it is nevertheless reasonable to draw a line there. This follows from the conjunction of three things. First, it is reasonable to distinguish in some way unacceptable cases from acceptable cases; second, the only way of doing that in these circumstances is to draw a sharp line; third, it cannot be an objection to drawing the line just here that it would have been no worse to draw it somewhere else – if that were an objection, then one could conclude that one had no reason to draw it anywhere, and that is a style of argument that led to the death of Buridan's ass, who (it will be remembered) died of starvation between two piles of hay because neither pile had any characteristic that drew him to it rather than to the other.

A line such as Warnock proposes may be unreasonable on some other grounds, but it is not so merely because it is this kind of line. Whether it will be effective is another question. If it is less effective than the alternative of allowing no cases at all, that will be because of the special circumstances such as those in which there is a consensus of allowing no cases, if that is all that can be achieved, but there is no consensus for anything else. Equally familiar, on the other hand, is a situation in which there is a consensus for allowing something rather than nothing, and a further consensus gradually emerges about what is to be allowed – a consensus, perhaps, formed as a result of recommending or legislating just such a line.

On this account, the slippery slope argument should be properly understood as in good part an empirical, consequentialist, argument. It does of course assume certain evaluations; in the present case, all parties are assuming that experimentation on a neonate would be unacceptable. It also has to make various judgements about what would be reasonable or equitable discriminations to make. But at the end of the line the argument is about what sort of social practice will in fact follow from adopting what kind of rule, and this is in good part an empirical argument. Many of the consequences to be considered will no doubt be of the kind that utilitarians are particularly concerned with, consequences for utility or welfare. But of course the consequences can be evaluated in other ways as well, for instance with respect to rights. The considerations about rights, if they are brought into the argument at this point, will not themselves be consequentialist arguments; but the slippery slope argument will itself be a consequentialist argument, to the general effect that if a certain rule is adopted or a certain practice allowed, then social consequences will follow in which (among other things) people's rights may be violated.

Seen in this light, it seems to me that the slippery slope style of argument can carry weight, and is to be taken seriously; but that, equally, it need not necessarily carry the day, in the sense of proving that the first step should never be taken. We may, instead, take the Warnock path of drawing a line, and that is a perfectly reasonable reaction, in the right circumstances, to the challenge that is indeed posed by the slippery slope considerations.

Some people, however, feel that this level of argument is too superficial to deal with the kind of ethical problem posed by embryo experimentation. They seek some 'absolute' consideration that will clearly settle the issue without invoking this sort of argument at all. Thus some people feel that they are on stronger ground if they say straightforwardly that the embryo is from the beginning a human being, and we should not kill or experiment on any human being (or, with regard to killing, at least on any innocent human being: there are various casuistical complications at this point which we can leave aside). This may be called the *definitional* approach. It looks different from the sort of thing that I have so far been discussing, and, as I have said, some people think that it is more solid and robust. But I think that this impression is an illusion, and in the last part of my remarks I shall try to show that inasmuch as this approach has any rationale, it is one that itself rests on the slippery slope argument – indeed, on two separate applications of it.

An embryo which, if all goes well, will develop into a human being is certainly a human embryo, but that does not imply that it is itself a human being. Those who insist that it is, make a great deal of its potentiality for normal development into a human being, thus distinguishing it from an ovum or a spermatozoon (which may be human but is not a human being). But in general this is not a natural way to describe or think of items which in the normal course of events have the potentiality of developing into a mature form that belongs to a given species. We do not naturally regard viable acorns as oak trees, or caterpillars as butterflies, and, as Jonathan Glover said in a televised debate, his opponent would be put out if, having been invited to a chicken dinner, he were served with an omelette made of fertilized eggs. This rather brutal joke outraged his opponent, but it made an entirely valid point.

More immediate and obviously significant than these general points is the fact that women do not regard an early embryo in the same light as a neonate or a fully developed foetus. Their experience of miscarriage can take many different forms, and for some, no doubt, an early miscarriage can be almost as traumatic as stillbirth. But it does not have to be, and it would be a cruel impertinence for some metaphysician to insist that the loss involved in each of these things had to be equivalent.

It is thus not true to our experience, with regard to human birth, or more generally, that the embryo has to be seen as a human being, and there is much in our experience to make natural the description that many would give, that the embryo is something that develops into a human being. So what basis is there for insisting that, despite these appearances, it must be a human being? The insistence may, of course, be based merely on supposed supernatural revelation. But if not, I suspect that it comes from an argument something like the following:

(1) 'Human being' is an absolute term.
(2) Development is a gradual process.
(3) Development ends in a human being.
(4) If development starts with a non-human being, there must be a cut-off point.
(5) Any cut-off point is arbitrary.
(6) There cannot be an arbitrary cut-off point.
Therefore, development must start with a human being.

This is itself a slippery slope argument, of what I called earlier the *arbitrary result* kind. The idea behind it is that since 'human being' is an absolute term – that is to say, nothing is more or less of a human being – it must be unacceptable to have a situation in which there is no definite starting point to something's being a human being, or only an arbitrary imposed starting point. But from a purely logical or semantic point of view, there is no reason to accept this. Very many terms, such as the names of many artifacts, are 'absolute' in this sense, but no one would insist on imposing a definite moment for the start of their being the sort of thing that they come to be.

In the previous argument, we can certainly accept premisses (5) and (6), while premisses (1), (2), and (3) are indisputable. The implausible premiss is (4), and without this, of course, the *arbitrary result* slippery slope argument will not work. Why should anyone accept (4)? It is certainly not imposed on us by purely logical or semantic argument. The reason, I suspect, actually lies in another slippery slope argument, this time of the *horrible result* kind: namely, that unless some definite point is imposed, we shall have a slippery slope that ends up with the horrible practice of experimentation on neonates.

The definitional approach, then, seems either to be quite arbitrary in its assumptions, or else to rely on the superimposition of one slippery slope on another: in the form of an *arbitrary result* argument, it presses the results of a linguistic practice which is itself only motivated by a *horrible result* argument.

The definitional approach has at least two disadvantages. One is that it fails to reveal what its real basis is: if slippery slope arguments are to be used sensibly on these matters, then a first requirement is that they should be recognized for what they are. The second disadvantage is that if people insist that the early embryo is a human being, this may produce results quite different from those that they want. It is as likely, or indeed more likely, that the result will be, not to suppress all experiments on embryos, but to admit an exception to the rule that human beings should not be killed for medical purposes or experimented on without their consent. If exceptions are admitted to the rule, we shall certainly be confronted with a slippery slope – one more threatening than those already considered.

References

Warnock, M. (1985) *A Question of Life*. Oxford: Basil Blackwell
Williams, B. (1986) What slopes are slippery? In M. Lockwood (ed.)
    Moral Dilemmas in Modern Medicine. Oxford University Press

Discussion/General Discussion

The slippery slope

Clothier: Have the scientists here, in embarking on interesting lines of research, ever felt that they had not only got onto the slippery slope but had slid down it into something terrible? Have you ever realized you were going too fast down such a slope? We must try to make some recommendations before we end this meeting.

Johnson: The slippery slope argument must also have underlain much of the debate and concern about evolutionary theory and whether there was a particular moment at which the human race came into being. Does the way in which religions have resolved that theological problem shed any useful light on the question before us now?

Williams: Our knowledge of the earlier hominid species is very patchy. There is of course a greater difference between one species and another, on the whole, than there is between one day's development of an embryo and the next day's development. Of course, if you have a picture that there is an absolute distinction between being a full-blown ensouled human being and something that is nothing of the kind, you will have a problem equally with phylogeny and ontogeny. The idea that you are either just a machine or a full-blown rational intelligence is, in traditional philosophical terms, only one idea among many others. It is certainly not the Aristotelian view of life, for instance, in which being ensouled is something that all living things have in different forms, depending on the type of life that each thing leads.

Edwards: The danger of drawing a line is that it may have to be modified later. Once the line is drawn, there could be far more difficulty in modifying it than if it had not been drawn in the first place. What we need is a braking system.

In relation to Warnock, I believe a better alternative to the fourteen-day rule is to establish a powerful ethical authority which demands justification for every piece of research. The fourteen-day rule is too generous for some research; for example the study of chromosomes can largely (but not entirely) be done at day five. Studies on the differentiation of the haemopoietic system would require embryos at day fourteen or perhaps later. For the myocardium it would be necessary to go to day twenty. Each of these is a legitimate study, yet if an arbitrary line is drawn some of them are excluded.

Williams: That is equally true if you want to study the development of intelligence, for instance; if you want to discover the neurological effects of socialization on the brain, five years is a good age. But people object to these experiments and they need reassurance. The argument that something would be an interesting experiment is not adequate.

The body to which you refer would have to be not only a technical body but also an ethical body. An ethical body has to carry authority, but there is no ethical body that carries authority in this sense in a pluralistic society. There aren't any experts on ethical knowledge. Why should anyone trust such a body? Drawing a line is the only fundamental way of reassuring people in the face of a genuine slippery slope argument. The more that medical researchers say it would be very interesting to do more experiments later, the less reassured the public will be, and the more need there is for a line. I agree with you that it is difficult to change the line – that is part of its point – but it is not unchangeable. Your objection to this line seems to be that it makes things slightly more difficult for your colleagues: but that is what it is for.

Edwards: My objection is that a line cannot cope with every situation.

Williams: The rule says 'at most fourteen days', not that every experiment has to go on until fourteen days. Your objection can only be that there are some other things you want to do after fourteen days.

Edwards: There are no ethical grounds for placing the limit further than is needed for a particular piece of work. An arbitrary fourteen-day rule would allow some scientists to let embryos grow for too long, in order to get certain answers. One rule of embryo research must be to terminate the stage of growth as early as possible. If a result can be obtained at day one, then stop at day one. A fourteen-day rule would be too generous in this respect.

Clothier: You want *ad hoc* decisions for everything, but propagating *ad hoc* decisions and enabling people to plan their activities is extremely difficult. The main thing about a rule is that it is the lowest common denominator to which everyone can subscribe, and at least it gives some sort of certainty.

Bowker: In practice, how are we going to live together? Rule-making is one way in which we get a consensus on where we will draw a line.

The slippery slope question asks, where is the soul, or when does it appear? However, you might prefer to talk about emergent properties. We all know the difference between a hill and a mountain, but what about the foothills? Are they hills or mountains? This is how I think religion got involved in animation and ensoulment. The anthropologists in the 1950s were on this slope when they discussed the cerebral rubicon and at what point the evolutionary process took a line of evolution over some threshold.

A Roman Catholic view

Iglesias: My view of Bernard Williams' slippery slope is that one should not get onto the slope – on the principle that we should not deliberately damage or destroy a harmless human life, or a human being, or whatever other name we want to give it. That has been the tradition of the Roman Catholic religion for 2000 years. By 'tradition' I mean the attitudes and authoritative teaching of the Church, not just theological discussion. This teaching is quite clear-cut, compared with the diverse response of other religions that Professor Bowker described.

I share with Professor Williams the view that the term 'human being' is an absolute term. Thus, what begins at conception is either a human being or isn't. But Bernard Williams thinks that the early embryo is not a human being and I think it is. How would I establish my position? First by tackling the reasons why Professor Williams thinks the embryo *is not* a human being, which have not been given. Then I would say that a human being does not come into existence in instalments, or brick by brick as a house does; it must come into being as an organic whole. And the time it does this is at conception.

Another point. If one recognizes the early embryo as a human being it is because one participates in a whole *form of life* which permits one to see human beings and their personal history in certain ways. Reasons and arguments will not easily affect another's form of life, as we well know: life precedes reasons. A form of life is primarily a *vision lived*; it is not ultimately founded on mere reasons. That is why Wittgenstein very wisely said in his book *On Certainty*: 'At the end of reasons comes persuasion'.

I do not hold the view that one can belong to humankind as a biological being without possessing a spiritual soul; nor do I think that the soul is an entity that comes to the biological being some time after conception. This is bad philosophy. The soul, if anything, is the principle of life, so by definition if a human organism is alive it is a human 'ensouled' being.

My approach to this question of full humanness is not explicitly in terms of the soul. What we must consider is the significance we attach to the human being generated at conception because of the kind of being it actually is and what it does and the potentialities it actually possesses. Also, we must consider why some people don't attach full human significance to those early stages of our development. Here there are two issues. One is the moral principle: do we get onto the slippery slope at all? Do we adhere to the view that we can deliberately harm and destroy beings of humankind for the benefit of others? To this I would say no. The second issue is, what counts as a human being? I would tackle this question, as I said before, by considering the reasons why the early human embryo is thought not to be a human being and the weight, either scientific or philosophical, which those reasons have.

Clothier: Is the oocyte a human being?

Iglesias: I would say that the human being is the newly formed conceptus after fertilization when a living organism or a living being of humankind has been generated as a whole.

Clothier: So it is a human being as soon as the sperm penetrates the egg?

Iglesias: As soon as the process of fertilization is completed, so that the conceptus is formed.

Williams: You made two points in favour of your way of looking at it. One is a metaphysical or logical point, namely that 'human being' is an on/off term. That grammatical fact is a very poor basis for the argument that a human being can't come from something that isn't a human being. This grammatical fact is a feature shared by something such as a tree or a building or a town hall. You can't be more or less of a town hall or more or less of a tree, for the same grammatical reason. That doesn't mean that the tree can't come from something that isn't a tree or that a town hall can't come from a pile of bricks.

A much deeper argument is drawn from the form of life; that is, we naturally see human beings in certain ways. You may be deceiving yourself about this argument, though, because we don't see things altogether in this way. We do not see fertilized eggs, larval stages, and so on as exactly the equivalent of adults. This applies to human beings: relevant reactions are to be found in the experience of women having miscarriages, stillbirths, and so on. If you go down to the deepest basis of human experience and try to discover it from that picture, you won't get the result that you and your church want, Dr Iglesias. Similarly, when the church tries to introduce a ban on birth control for metaphysical/theological reasons, the experience of life of a very large number of sincere Catholics makes them vote with their feet. The ban does not express the form of life that they actually live.

Harper: I think that the official Catholic view of when life begins is relatively recent, dating from when the church had to codify its official position and write it down, rather than representing a 2000-year tradition, as was claimed. Unlike other religions the Catholic church has views on infallibility and unchangeability so it can't get itself out of what others see as an illogical position. Much of the argument that goes on attempts to square the circle and doesn't have any very long-standing basis in Catholic or Christian tradition at all.

Iglesias: Many people recognize that a human life should not be destroyed or harmed for the benefit of others. You do not need a particular religion and a particular creed of faith to hold to that principle of natural justice. Nevertheless this principle has been defended by the Catholic church's authoritative teaching body, the bishops, throughout the centuries. Some theologians might discuss this question now but neither at present nor in the past have the body of bishops and the church as a whole ever objected to or abandoned the view that innocent human life should not be deliberately harmed or destroyed from the beginning of its existence at conception.

Casey: A human being is an absolute being in the sense that one cannot say one is partly a human being, but in another sense this is a concept with fuzzy boundaries. We recognize underlying similarities in some group of objects or beings and we apply a name to those which are sufficiently similar, be they 'human beings' or 'tables'. Nevertheless if something is sticking out of the wall I may well argue about whether it is a table or a shelf. Unless for some purpose you deliberately adopt a very tight definition, any concept will have a fuzzy boundary to it. An acorn grows into an oak tree, but there is some point in between at which you may not be sure whether you should yet dignify it with the name of tree.

Also, one may regard X as being Y for a particular purpose. So a lawyer (perhaps speaking loosely) may say that a company is 'a person' in law. What the lawyer means is that for that particular purpose a company has an important characteristic in common with what we all understand as a person (in this case that it can sue and be sued). Similarly, if we say that 'the conceptus is a human being' we are either *defining* human being more widely than normal language does, or saying that in our view, for a particular purpose, it shares some important relevant characteristic with the things that everyone calls human beings. In that case it may be useful to ask what those who take this view believe that characteristic is.

Dunstan: As a Church of England man I sometimes consider it my duty to spring to the defence of the Roman Catholic church. I do so at this moment because it is not true that the position of the Roman Catholic church is as uniform as it is sometimes represented to be. Gregory of Nyssa, St Augustine, and Pope Innocent III were all bishops of the Catholic church and none of them would accept some of the propositions made by Dr Iglesias today. There is a long historical tradition behind the conjunction of the Aristotelian concept of animation and the Hippocratic understanding of morphology. The *Journal of Medical Ethics* for March 1984 has a very clear account of one philosophical position (Iglesias 1984) and an accurate exposition of the Western moral tradition on the moral status of the human embryo (Dunstan 1984). As Professor

Harper suggested, the present authoritative teaching of the Roman Catholic church is in strict truth a novelty. Its present form dates from 1869.

Another fact is that among contemporary Catholic teachers Dr Iglesias's position would not be upheld. The book by Dr John Mahoney, S.J., *Bioethics and Belief* (Mahoney 1984) expounds an approach to *in vitro* fertilization which seeks to take account of the facts of the case as he understands them and of the moral tradition which I have alluded to. Dr Mahoney has certainly not come to the same conclusion as Teresa Iglesias. Her position may be defensible but I do not believe that it is the uniform position of the Roman Catholic church, or ever has been.

Iglesias: The official teaching authority of the Catholic church has always been the bishops in communion with the Pope, not just a single theologian or number of theologians. The document on *Procured Abortion* (Sacred Congregation 1974) that was ratified by Pope Paul VI states that the principle that human life from conception is not to be deliberately destroyed or harmed represents a Christian view and attitude that has never changed and is unchangeable. In that sense I would say that the Catholic tradition has been uniform. This is not my personal view only; a scholarly historical work on the subject by John Connery, S.J., entitled *Abortion: The Development of the Roman Catholic Perspective* (1977), makes this same point clearly.

Dunstan: The question was at what point in its development the embryo acquires such a human status that its destruction becomes homicide. The equation of that point with conception was not made until 1869.

Towards a consensus

Rodeck: It would be a great help if we separated destruction of human life (implying wantonness) from destruction carried out for the advancement of potentially beneficial knowledge (with the implication of sacrifice). Sacrifice is something that the Christian religion apparently approves of. Christ and the saints died and sacrificed themselves. People who donate their kidneys are making a sacrifice too. The phrase used in American scientific journals, 'and the animals were sacrificed', which has often been mocked, may be touching on an important point.

Iglesias: If you are attacked unjustly you can defend yourself and you might cause the death of your attacker. This has always been defended as a principle as it has existed in practice, and as it is upheld by our laws. Yet the life of a harmless person must not be taken. You may even love your neighbour to the point of giving your life for him or her, but it is never morally permissible for you to take a person's life.

Bowker: There are particular procedures within any society for trying to reach some sort of consensus. An example of that would be how the Roman Catholic church has moved toward the concept of collegiality, in the way the bishops move towards the laity – at least in theory. This can produce a consensus with a degree of novelty within it. An example of new insight being brought to bear on old principles would be how to determine when a marriage hasn't happened. We now understand more clearly that there may be psychological reasons, not just physiological reasons, for non-consummation. Therefore there has been a considerable debate on the notion of psychological nullity. New insight gets locked onto the existing debate and principles, without any denial of the concept of nullity. I wouldn't want to say whether that is wise.

So there are principles within the Christian tradition which could and should be brought to bear on this discussion. In the past they have not been brought in, largely because this is an unprecedented situation. Since we are part of a process of trying to form a consensus, it is extremely important not to let that point go by. One of the purposes of a group of this kind is to try to draw attention to those new principles, or to old principles being brought to bear on new situations.

Maddox: It would be helpful if we looked at other circum-stances where there is a consensus on the preservation of human life. For example we all agree that we should not kill each other at the older end of the spectrum. People have talked about euthanasia for a very long time but have shrunk away from it, recognizing it to be a slippery slope leading to horrible results. At the other end it is interesting that courts are very lenient in sentencing people convicted of maternal infanticide. It is surprising how much infanticide happens in hospitals when an infant is trisomic (has Down's syndrome) and so on. There is a consensus in this country in favour of controlled abortion up to about twenty-eight weeks. Society accepts that the degree to which a mother has got attached to her unborn foetus is the determining factor. If we follow that line, we are not going to be able to sustain the argument that embryos are human beings to whom we owe the same duty of protection.

Fertilization of donated oocytes for research

McLaren: There have been several references to the creation of embryos for research. This is a misleading phrase. 'Creation' of course has theological connotations. Also, as we discussed earlier, embryo is an ambiguous term. What actually happens is that women who come in for sterilization by tubal ligation are asked whether they would be prepared to donate oocytes to be fertilized for research purposes. Quite a high proportion of women are happy to do this. That rings true to me. It is the end of one's own reproductive life and all those eggs in one's ovaries are going to waste. If they can be used to help infertile couples or prevent genetic defects that is an act of generosity, not a sacrifice.

   Much of the research on such oocytes is concerned with the act of fertilization itself and with the early cleavage that follows. Research on fertilization can only be done on material of that sort. It can't be done on spare embryos that have been fertilized for therapeutic purposes. It might be worth discussing the ethical aspects of this.

Clothier: That research differs from the fertilization of eggs

taken for the purposes of *in vitro* fertilization because for
IVF you try to ensure a pregnancy by taking more than
you need, and you end up with a surplus.

McLaren: In IVF all the eggs are fertilized for therapeutic
purposes and it would be unethical to experiment on them
in any way. The eggs that had been experimented on
might later be needed in the course of therapy.

Clothier: Professor Edwards said that he takes more eggs than
most people because he doesn't see any point in not taking
them.

Braude: He made the point clearly that we cannot decide, at the
present stage of our knowledge, which of those oocytes
are going to fertilize. The priority is to achieve a
pregnancy for the patient. If we could store oocytes in
such a way that we could fertilize them on request it
would be different, but we cannot do that yet.

McLaren: Those techniques of oocyte storage are not going to be
developed unless it is possible to do research on donated
oocytes.

Hull: The comparison between human and mouse embryos is
confused. Certain special values are attached to the human
embryo and we are faced with semantic problems. It
bothers me that Dr Iglesias refers to innocent life. 'Life', as
she uses the word, implies being, as in a person, and is not
distinguished from being alive. Innocence is a state which
requires consciousness or at the very least sentience, and
that cannot apply to the early human embryo. To me the
early embryo does not have any special value and
therefore it doesn't matter whether embryos are made
especially for research. What matters is the purpose of
that research. It would be absolutely wrong to undertake
research with the danger of creating a monster that might
be born.

Another ethical point is that you mustn't do something
that puts the woman who is donating an egg at special risk.
Anne McLaren has explained how to avoid that. There are
other more general issues about research. We shouldn't
undertake any sort of research, even if it only produces
discomfort, if we don't end up with a scientifically valid
answer. But to return to the fundamental issue, I would

wish that we could come to a decision that it was neither evil nor good to deal with the early embryo.

Braude: Both of these arguments come down to the point of view that we have to establish the moral status of the early preimplantation embryo. At the moment there seems to be an assumption that this deserves respect in a particular way. The only person who has come clean is John Maddox, who said that he doesn't believe it has a moral status at that time. In general, society also doesn't believe it has a special moral status. Society is quite prepared to use postcoital contraception such as the intrauterine contraceptive device and kill off preimplantation embryos. Very few people get up in arms about this.

Baird: When you went to Oldham to collect eggs in 1970, was it your intention to put these fertilized embryos back in that woman, Professor Edwards?

Edwards: When we went to Oldham before 1970, there was no research at all on the human embryo. It was our intention to establish a programme for the replacement of embryos. The patients giving oocytes were infertile and might have benefited from this work. We had to grow some embryos from these patients in order to see whether they developed to the blastocyst stage and whether their chromosomes were normal. I accept that that was a pure research period but it has now passed. Since then numerous embryos have been replaced and many pregnancies have been established. There are now tissues from abnormal embryos *in vitro* that could be used for research, as Peter Braude described. Such research could use those with three pronuclei, which are possible triploid embryos, which arise accidentally and could not be replaced in the mother. The decision to use such abnormal embryos is one that should be referred to the scientists or the doctors. But to establish embryos for research is a very different matter.

Baird: So you felt at that time that the question was sufficiently important to justify collecting eggs and fertilizing them, even though that would compromise the life of that particular embryo?

Edwards: Yes, that was so at that time.

Is there an ethical distinction?

Clothier: If you have consent from the donor or the creator of the eggs to start with, it may be conditional for 'spare' embryos and absolute for embryos donated for research. Donors can say 'I'll give these to you on condition that you give them back if you successfully fertilize them' or 'You can have them because they are no longer any use to me'. If you have the consent in both cases, what is the ethical distinction which worries you?

McLaren: This is what I hoped we would clarify.

Williamson: I feel this dilemma too. If Bob Edwards has some fertilized eggs left over that he is going to throw away I can see no difficulty in using these for research. I feel much more reluctance, but I am not clear why, about taking an oocyte from someone who has been sterilized and fertilizing it for research.

Baird: I find that view very difficult to understand. Those who have ethical objections to experimenting on embryos have them for the sake of the embryo. They don't consider that the person who is giving informed consent for their egg or their embryo to be experimented on has the right to interfere with that individual embryo. If that is the premiss on which there is an objection to experimenting on embryos, I can see no difference, from the embryo's point of view, between whether it is brought into being for the purpose of being experimented on or whether it happens to be surplus to requirements for therapeutic purposes.

Williamson: The premiss might be more along the lines that it is inherently wasteful to throw something away which could otherwise be made good use of in humanitarian terms. In the same way, when you switch off a life-support machine it is inherently wasteful not to make every attempt to use the kidneys and any other organs that one can. Creating something in order to do these things seems to me to be different. It is not based on any particular view of the rights of the embryo.

McLaren: If I was being sterilized I would feel it was inherently wasteful for the oocytes not to be used if they could be.

Edwards: The reason why we have never been keen on research embryos is based first on the intent of the research worker. I am fully prepared to agree that if we had thousands of human embryos *in vitro* we would get some excellent results. If the decision to accept research embryos is ever taken by Parliament or any other authority, I would take advantage of it.

Dunstan: When the question about spare embryos and those created for research was put to me earlier [Chapter 5, discussion] I deliberately diverted it to Anthony Dyson so that he could expand his minority statement in the Warnock Report (1984, p. 94), where he opposed the creation of embryos *ad hoc* for research purposes. My own view is somewhat different but has no finality attached to it. I am all the time thinking my way through this.

First, the distinction between using spare embryos and creating them for research purposes is one where what I believe to be a false antithesis rests on *nefas*, O horror! This, I think, is Bob Williamson's condition. He feels this to be wrong but he has yet to find a reason why it should be wrong. Discussions about contraception and analgesia in childbirth have a long negative history of this sort too. Our initial gut reaction is not a final moral judgement. By a process of moral reasoning we have to form moral judgements on our gut reactions. This is what I try to do. I would distinguish between creating an entity called an embryo, to which we may or may not attach a particular status, and initiating or furthering a process. All that has been said by the scientists here would indicate that the second way is the better way of talking about what you are doing. You are initiating or furthering a process in which changes happen.

The word intention has been brought into this. The intention of someone who puts spermatozoa and oocytes together is to further that process. The intention is fulfilled in the resulting action. But the intention is not the last word. That intention must be directed towards a purpose and I suspect that the moral significance attaches more to the end or purpose of the act than to the intention in performing the act. The purposes for which this process is initiated may be diverse. They may be directly intended to remedy infertility in one particular woman who has given the oocyte and her husband who has given the sperm. In an area of developing medical practice there is a diversity of purposes around that. The people who want to use embryos for other related purposes do so, I think, on this ground: the remedying of one woman's infertility is a special case of providing remedies for infertility in general. One area of infertility surrounds deficiencies in male sperm, for example, and the testing of sperm on oocytes may be the only way to find out. We can imagine a variety of purposes for which this process is related to the remedy of infertility in a sense of achieving healthy viable babies, in which one particular baby is a special case. A procedure adopted for one particular case may be extended beyond the individual to a cluster of individuals who are at present anonymous but who all become living persons with living human interests when they arrive at a clinic one by one with their problems.

The second stage in the argument is this. Our discussions have shown that these purposes cannot all be achieved by the use of spare embryos alone. The embryos that are not put back into the mother are presumed to be less good than those which were put back. We cannot assume therefore that they are typical of normal embryonic development. And as freezing techniques improve there will be fewer embryos left 'spare', because they will be frozen. Again, for some purposes you cannot operate experimentally on already fertilized oocytes. For practical reasons you cannot achieve a good end or good purpose by using spares alone. By the time it has been decided which embryos *are* spare, the period for some critical observations has already passed. Therefore, if your aim is to show your respect for the sanctity of life, however manifested and from its earliest time onwards, and if you want to show this respect by economy, let us say by never using more embryos than you must and using every one respectfully and for a legitimate purpose, then you may achieve this economic aim more quickly by doing specific, controlled experiments on oocytes fertilized for your purposes, than by tying yourself to material available by chance, working randomly on spares left over because they are inadequate for the original purpose. Good research might well reduce the number of implanted embryos needed to secure a pregnancy, and so reduce the need to superovulate for multiple oocytes. If you add the question of purpose to the concept of intent, and if you enlarge that purpose to such an extent that you include the general case as well as the particular, and if one aspiration is towards economy in the disposal of embryonic life, out of respect for it, I myself could not say that the creation of embryos *ad hoc* is morally illicit; if we accept research on 'spares' we can accept the others also. The proper distinction should be between embryos destined for maturity in the womb, and assessed for adequacy as such, and those destined for related research: embryos either inadequate in themselves, or marred by observation or experiment, should not be reimplanted in the uterus.

Edwards: This debate is about fertilizing eggs, taking a decision to establish an embryo that has no chance of survival because it will never be replaced in the mother. The intent is to establish it, and then use it for research.

Dunstan: Death is a consequence, not the intent.

Edwards: The consequence lies in the intent. Society should make such decisions. Another similar problem concerns the decision not to go beyond day fourteen. This is another scientific argument, just as with spare embryos. Many reasons can be put forward as to why we should grow an embryo beyond day fourteen. Likewise, if embryos were placed in a chimpanzee they might grow to beautiful blastocysts. That has not been done. Now that the gamete intra-Fallopian transfer (GIFT) technique has been introduced, unfertilized eggs and sperm could be put in the human oviduct and embryos could be grown *in utero* for research. There are all types of work with ethical overtones that might be done, besides establishing research embryos, but they are not done. Geoffrey

Hawthorn and Bernard Williams pointed out that public morality limits what we can do.

In my view the triploid embryo grows equally well as a diploid to a blastocyst and I do not agree with Peter Braude that it has no value in research. It is a material that is suitable for work such as he described and we can use it without challenging these fundamental tenets about research embryos while those tenets are being decided. It is wise for scientists to proceed slowly and to raise these issues for wide debate, until Parliament or some delegated authority decides them. The debate is now widespread and involves Parliament; this was not so in 1970. If we raise these issues for debate we show that we are concerned about them. The public attitude towards science is difficult enough already without going ahead irrespective of other people's views.

Gerard: To my surprise, I found myself in total agreement with Professor Dunstan when he said that, provided scientists produce the results quickly, it doesn't really matter whether one uses spare embryos or deliberately created ones. It is the time limit which is of overwhelming importance.

Building a framework

Modell: Is the conclusion the chairman would like us to reach concerned with a time limit, or also with the ethical issue of whether embryos should be created specifically for research or whether embryos created for other purposes should be used?

Clothier: There should eventually be some outcome of value to practical scientists. The meeting should enable us all to go our various ways and then contribute to the establishment of rules which will be generally acceptable to the greatest number of people. We need to make a framework within which we can live together and work together without running into animosities. This meeting has no authority to lay down rules.

Modell: I did have reservations about the fertilization of donated ova until I heard the discussion. Now they have been resolved, primarily by Anne McLaren's remarks.

At a recent meeting of the World Health Organisation's Advisory Group on Hereditary Disease we were asked to discuss the ethical aspects of present practices in genetics, partly because of the potential for widespread anxiety that can be raised by minority groups. We felt that people became anxious partly because they did not know or fully understand how clinical genetics is practised, and we thought that a professional code of conduct might remove much of this anxiety. In particular, people are disturbed by the idea that governments might use these techniques for unethical purposes.

To begin with, we agreed the statement of principle, that 'The objective of the genetics services is to help people with a genetic disadvantage to live and to reproduce as normally and responsibly as possible.'

The proposed code is not concerned with research but I feel it has some relevance to our topic. Core principles in the code are the autonomy of the individual or the couple, their right to adequate and complete information, and the maintenance of the highest standards of confidentiality. These principles are in fact adhered to in genetics practice: it follows that each case is treated as a separate entity in its individual context, and not in relation to the previous couple or case. In real clinical practice, the slippery slope doesn't exist.

References

Connery, J. (1977) *Abortion: The Development of the Roman Catholic Perspective*. Chicago: Loyola University Press

Dunstan, G.R. (1984) The moral status of the human embryo: a tradition recalled. *Journal of Medical Ethics* 10: 38–44

Iglesias, T. (1984) *In vitro* fertilisation: the major issues. *Journal of Medical Ethics* 10: 32–7

Mahoney, J. (1984) *Bioethics and Belief*. London: Sheed and Ward, Ch. 1 and 3

Sacred Congregation (1974) Declaration by the Sacred Congregation for the Doctrine of the Faith on Procured Abortion, Rome, 18 November 1974. [English version: Catholic Truth Society, London, 1974]

Warnock, M. (Chairman) (1984) *Report of the Committee of Inquiry into Human Fertilisation and Embryology*. London: HMSO (Department of Health & Social Security) Cmnd. 9314

THIRTEEN

Conclusion

Sir Cecil Clothier

We began this meeting with a brilliant exposition by Dr McLaren of what happens at the start of reproduction, which provided a model around which the entire symposium has been able to revolve. Armed with that information we moved into the phase of seeing what could be done to better the lot of the human race if research on early human embryos was permissible within limits which have yet to be determined. We immediately identified five areas which were extremely important and capable of furtherance by research into early human embryos: the diagnosis and treatment of infertility, its relief by *in vitro* fertilization, the diagnosis of genetic disease, the causes and avoidance of congenital malformations, and the improvement of contraception.

I imagine there will be very little dispute that those are all worthy objects of research because they confer great benefits on the human race. Whether the list is five or 500 none of these areas of research would be justified if what is proposed to be done is ethically unacceptable. All we have done is to make a case for doing the research. Obviously that is essential or the rest of the argument is superfluous. If we establish that there are misfortunes in humanity which may be relieved in this way the first step has been taken towards seeking to justify it.

The central problem is the determination of the point in a cycle at which a group of cells is entitled to a special regard, or to some sort of rights. Alternatively, at what point do we owe that group a special duty? I think that rights are as important as duties and are not to be disregarded. They are the reciprocals of duty. These things are a unity, not two separate concepts. Whichever way you look at it, there obviously comes a moment when the development of the cells that could ultimately form a human being require us to give them some special attention in the form of a protection on which we all agree.

I have an uncomfortable feeling that the lawyers and philosophers have let the scientists down. We haven't produced a set of rules which would satisfy everyone as to what is permissible and what is not, that could be used as a yardstick in an area where science is moving at a tremendous rate. The whole concept on which we have all been proceeding is that life began at some point in space and then proceeded along a linear track until it became a recognizable human being. But we are wrong. It is not a linear notion but a circular notion; and it is more arbitrary to break into a circle than to break into a line. If you break into a circle you may get back to where you started. Nevertheless plainly we will have to choose in the end an arbitrary moment in the cycle and say that the duty of preservation and non-interference arises at that moment. Alternatively we have to say that that cluster of cells has a right to integrity from that point onwards on the circle or on the line.

There was after all something to be said for the old-fashioned lawyer's phrases 'quick with child' and 'life in being'. They had the virtues of simplicity and certainty. One knew when 'quickness' was happening and when the life was capable of being sustained apart from the mother, or one believed one did. One didn't need to be a scientist to observe them. So maybe it is the scientists who have let the lawyers down by being too clever by half. You have presented us with the most frightful problems and confused us beyond belief. We thought we knew when we had a human being whom we had to respect as such and who was recognizable as such. By going further and further back along the chain of particle coalescence you have shown us that we were talking nonsense. I just wonder whether we were; but you have landed us with a problem which I don't think lawyers will be able to solve easily. I don't suppose we thought this symposium would produce answers to these immensely difficult questions but our discussions have certainly given us a basis of sound information and thinking on which to proceed to the next stage of helping the man on the Clapham omnibus, who has not been thinking about it very much, to come to an extremely important conclusion.

I am reminded of the county court judge who had the misfortune to have the awful F.E. Smith appearing before him. The judge was sufficiently imprudent to say 'After hearing your opening, Mr Smith, I'm afraid I am none the wiser.' 'Indeed you are not' came back the sharp reply, 'but you are a good deal better informed.' That is how I feel. I haven't grown any wiser but I feel much better able to discuss what should happen next and how and in what way we should formulate some rules which will both allay the proper anxieties of society and at the same time enable the search for the truth about human life to go forward properly.

The Warnock Report was criticized somewhat by Mr Hawthorn but on the whole it is a remarkably good document. The fourteen-day rule has something to be said for it: it is workable, it is observable, it has a quality of certainty about it — there is an important change at fourteen days.

After the scientific presentations it was time for the moral philosophers to come to our aid. The religious approach is one that I found difficult, maybe because thirty years as a lawyer makes one naturally sceptical of the most elementary assertions. I think Professor Bowker got very near to saying that there is not much point in establishing a reconciliation between religious philosophies of life and practical rules for the pursuit of knowledge. He mentioned that a doctor who may be a devout Hindu lives one religious life and a rather different medical life. That may be absolutely necessary for his sane existence.

On the other hand Bernard Williams convinced me that the slippery slope is not linear but has a very sharp climb at the start, followed by a flattening of the curve thereafter. This would be a new concept in Whitehall and would be welcomed if they got to know about it. Professor Williams reassured me in my belief that in the end you have to be arbitrary, you have to draw your line, look at it, and choose a place. That is true in pretty well all kinds of law making and rule making. In the end you have to choose a point which you think will cause the least trouble and draw the line there, where by and large it satisfies most people and allays the most anxieties. That was shown to be respectable from a quarter where authentication is very hard to find.

Glossary

allantois
a sac outside the embryo that in some mammals has an excretory and/or respiratory function, and in humans contributes to the formation of the umbilical cord

amnion
the membrane enclosing the embryo and the amniotic fluid in which the embryo develops

antibody
a protein synthesized by the body's white blood cells in response to an antigen

antigen
any substance that stimulates the formation of an antibody specific to that substance

biopsy
removal for examination of pieces of tissue from the living body

blastocyst
the hollow ball of cells resulting from cleavage of the zygote at the time of implantation in the uterine wall, before gastrulation. The blastocyst has an inner clump of cells (the inner cell mass) from which the embryo develops

chorionic villi
finger-like projections that develop from the chorion or outer membrane surrounding the embryo, amnion, and yolk sac, and that later help to form the placenta

codon
a triplet of nucleotides that forms the basic coding unit of DNA and determines the synthesis of a particular amino acid

corpus luteum	a glandular body that forms from the Graafian follicle of the ovary after extrusion of the ovum
diploid	having two sets of chromosomes, one from the mother and one from the father; twice the haploid number
DNA	deoxyribonucleic acid, the major constituent of the chromosomes, and the hereditary material of most living organisms
ectoderm	the outermost germ layer, q.v.
endoderm	the innermost germ layer, q.v.
endometriosis	a pathological condition in which the mucous membrane that normally lines the uterus is present in abnormal situations in the body
follicle	a group of cells forming a cavity or sheath. In the ovary the oocytes are surrounded by follicle cells; as the time of ovulation nears, a fluid-filled cavity appears in the follicle, which is now termed a Graafian follicle
fundus (of uterus)	the part of the uterus above the point of entry of the Fallopian tubes
gametes	the cells (spermatozoa and ova) which fuse to form a zygote in sexual reproduction
gastrulation	the stage during which the embryonic cells reorganize to form the germ layers
genome	the set of genes and chromosomes in any cell, organism, or species
genotype	the genetic complement of an organism (often contrasted with the phenotype, or appearance, of the organism)
germ layer	one of the three main layers of cells at the gastrulation stage of development, namely the ectoderm, mesoderm and endoderm, from which the various tissues and organs of the body are formed
gonadotropins	protein hormones that stimulate the gonads and regulate reproductive activity. Luteinizing hormone, follicle-stimulating

hormone and prolactin are pituitary gonadotropins present in both sexes. The presence of chorionic gonadotropin, secreted
by the chorionic villi of the placenta,
usually indicates pregnancy

haemoglobinopathy   a disease of the blood in which haemoglobin
in the red blood cells is abnormal

haploid   having the number of chromosomes characteristic of the gametes for the organism

hydatidiform mole   a pathological conceptus in which the
chorionic villi have undergone degener-
ation and which sometimes perforates the
wall of the uterus

inner cell mass   inner layer of the blastocyst from which the
embryo develops

karyotype   the chromosomal make-up; the appearance
of the set of chromosomes belonging to an
organism or cell, characteristic for each
species

laparoscopy   examination, under anaesthetic, of the ab-
dominal cavity with an illuminated
telescope-like instrument

maturation   in oocytes, the process that transforms the
primary oocyte into a mature gamete, the
ovum, ready to be fertilized

meiosis   process essential for the formation of the
gametes, by which a cell nucleus divides
into four nuclei, each with half the number
of chromosomes of the parent nucleus, after
segments of genetic material have been
exchanged between maternal and paternal
chromosome sets

mesoderm   the middle of the three germ layers, q.v.

morula   the clump of cells resulting from ovum
segmentation, before formation of the blastocyst, q.v.

neural tube   a tube formed after gastrulation that develops into the brain and spinal cord

oestrogens   steroid hormones, including oestradiol-17β

and oestrone, which stimulate the growth and maintenance of the female reproductive organs and affect reproductive function and behaviour

oncogene
a gene found in some viruses and thought to cause cancer

oocyte
a female cell that has entered meiosis (q.v.) but has not yet matured to form an ovum

ovum
a female gamete; egg

phenotype
the physical characteristics of an organism, determined by the genotype and the environment

polar body
the primary oocyte divides to form the polar body, a cell with very little cytoplasm, and a secondary oocyte, a cell with a large amount of cytoplasm that then divides into another polar body and an ovum. The polar bodies degenerate

polyploidy
the condition in which the basic (haploid) number of chromosomes is increased by more than twofold

pre-embryo
the conceptus from fertilization to the primitive streak stage (fifteen to eighteen days after ovulation in human females)

primitive streak
the longitudinal band of cells that forms a groove where germ layers are formed and the embryo begins to develop

progesterone
a steroid hormone produced mainly by the corpus luteum. Progesterone prepares the uterus to receive the fertilized egg and maintains the uterus during pregnancy

pronucleus
the egg or sperm nucleus after penetration of the egg by the sperm

RNA
ribonucleic acid, which occurs in cell cytoplasm and directs protein synthesis. Messenger RNA (mRNA) transfers the genetic information for protein synthesis from DNA to the ribosomes where protein synthesis takes place

testosterone	the main natural steroid hormone with masculinizing properties that is produced by the testis. It is also an intermediate in the biosynthesis of oestrogens
thalassaemia	a chronic and progressive form of inherited anaemia, occurring at high frequency in people from Mediterranean countries
transcription	the process by which the genetic information in a molecule of DNA is converted into a complementary strand of RNA, particularly messenger RNA
translation	a stage in protein synthesis in which the sequence of nucleotides in a molecule of messenger RNA is converted into a corresponding sequence of amino acids in a polypeptide chain
trisomy	having three chromosomes of one type instead of the normal two (e.g. trisomy 21, responsible for Down's syndrome)
trophectoderm	outer layer of the blastocyst; trophoblast
trophoblast	the layer of cells derived from the outer trophectoderm layer of the blastocyst
zona pellucida	the transparent glycoprotein membrane that surrounds the oocyte and is secreted by the ovarian follicle cells
zygote	cell formed by union of sperm and egg (reproductive cells)

Name index

Subject index

abortion 72, 73; availability, opinion polls 154, 155; in Hinduism 169; Islam and 173, 174; *in vitro* 78, 115; IVF, after 50, 56, 57; Judaism and 175

Abortion Act 1967 143

acetylcholine receptor genes 91

adenosine deaminase 95

allantois 11

Alzheimer's disease 110, 111

amenorrhoea 29, 31

amniocentesis 93, 94

amniotic cavity 11

animal *v*. human material in research 136, 137, 138, 139

ankyloglossia 108

antenatal diagnosis *see* prenatal diagnosis

anthropology 167, 170, 171, 180

anti-progestagen 123

anti-sperm antibodies 125, 127, 129, 130, 138

antithrombin III deficiency 88

anti-zona antibodies 125, 127, 129, 130

anti-zona vaccines 127, 129, 130

apolipoprotein genes 89

artificial insemination: donor 31, 34; husband 31

aryl-hydrocarbon hydroxalase 90

atman 167, 168, 171

autoimmune disease, genetic factors 84, 88

azoospermia 26, 29

Bhagavad Gita 170

bkm probe 102, 116

blastocyst 9, 10, 47, 72, 132, 133

blastocyst formation, timing of removal of cells for prenatal diagnosis and 10

blastocyst sexing 103

Brahman 167, 168, 170, 182, 183

Buddhism 166, 167, 171–73; aggregation in 171, 172; beginning of life and 172, 173; continuity in 171, 172; Japan, in 172, 173; pre-embryo research and 171, 172

Burkitt's lymphoma 90

232 *Human Embryo Research: Yes or No?*